To my mother, Kushma.

To my father, Hari.

To my sister, Nirvana, and brother, Ravi.

And especially to my daughter, Maya.

To Saraswati, the goddess of learning, art and wisdom.

Dr Nerina Ramlakhan

Fast Asleep, Wide Awake

Discover the Secrets of Restorative Sleep and Vibrant Energy

Thorsons

Thorsons
An imprint of HarperCollins*Publishers*
1 London Bridge Street
London SE1 9GF

www.harpercollins.co.uk

First published by Thorsons 2016

1 3 5 7 9 10 8 6 4 2

Text © Dr Nerina Ramlakhan 2016

Dr Nerina Ramlakhan asserts the moral right
to be identified as the author of this work

A catalogue record of this book is
available from the British Library

ISBN 978-0-00-817986-1

Printed and bound in Great Britain by
Clays Ltd, St Ives plc

MIX
Paper from
responsible sources

FSC
www.fsc.org   **FSC™ C007454**

FSC™ is a non-profit international organisation established to promote
the responsible management of the world's forests. Products carrying the
FSC label are independently certified to assure consumers that they come
from forests that are managed to meet the social, economic and
ecological needs of present and future generations,
and other controlled sources.

Find out more about HarperCollins and the environment at
www.harpercollins.co.uk/green

Contents

Acknowledgements

I am deeply grateful to all who provided the magic that made writing this book possible:

The clients and patients who have brought me so much insight and inspiration, and that little clinic in Moorgate where I first discovered the 'click' of doing the work I knew I was born to do.

All the people who have guided, supported and enabled me to bring the words through.

Sandy Draper, my editing doula – thank you for getting 'it' and me – and Carolyn Thorne at HarperCollins for her patience and belief in my message.

The special friends who understood my journey and have always supported just at the right time – Gosia Gorna, Nikola King, Luisa and Peter Diana-Kuramapu, Melanie Langer, Kerry-Lyn Stanton-Downes and Carolyn Kolasinski.

Lisa Lewisohn for her patience in putting up with the writing-induced mood swings.

And last but never least my daughter, Maya, for her great patience when I kept disappearing off to the shed to write.

Preface

'The unexamined life is not worth living.'

Plato

Last night I did something that I haven't been able to do for decades. I slept without my fan on.

It was 5 November, Bonfire Night, and the air crackled with light and colour. I could smell bonfires and hear distant sirens. Lying in bed I wondered if I'd be able to sleep and then I remembered that I hadn't turned on my fan. I have slept with a fan for many years – it acts as a buffer against the intrusion of noises out there and my own thoughts in here – but last night I decided I no longer needed it.

I slept deeply until morning, without any props.

I am called a sleep and energy expert. I've gained this reputation because I have a knack for solving people's sleep problems and I love doing this. But *even more* than this, I love helping people to live their lives with energy and meaning. I make no secret of the fact that my work stems from overcoming my own challenges with insomnia, but over the years I have learnt to sleep deeply and restoratively. And why? Because I have learnt how to deal with life head on.

Six years ago my first book, *Tired But Wired*, was published. As a result my career took off ... But I knew there was more to say. I began to see very clearly that while I was helping people to sleep, and the *Tired but Wired* Sleep Toolkit did this brilliantly, in doing so I was providing a bridge that took people to a place where they were able to deal with life with courage and resilience. And so I put pen to paper and began to write this book, which would help people to face life with all of its messiness and challenges – and thus *Fast Asleep, Wide Awake* was born.

Since starting to write this book over two years ago, a great deal has changed for me. You could say my life has been turned inside out. In 2013 my father died and then, just over two months ago, my 11-year marriage ended. For a time, it was enough to send me back to my old insomnia roots. Lying awake at night, unable to settle and turn off my mind. I put aside writing and gave my energies over to recalibrating my life. Two days ago I knew I was ready to resume work on this book. As I did so, the safety – which you'll discover is so fundamental to deep sleep – I had been reaching for, finally edged into view. Last night I arrived at a destination where I no longer needed the fan.

I know I'm not alone in facing cataclysmic changes in both my inner and outer worlds. Of late, life has been messy for many of us – I hear it on the news, witness it in my friends' lives and at my clinic, and see it in the corporate world where I speak to packed auditoriums where there's standing room only.

We need resilience and courage to do what I call the 'Real Work' of life. We need to sleep well so that we can heal and wake up with the energy and resources we need to face life with all of its disorder and challenges. By this I mean a certain type of sleep and a certain type of energy: sleep that is deep, pure and restorative, and vibrant energy that enables us to thrive – not just survive. I have learnt that to get this safe place we need to go deeper within ourselves, to find a peaceful stillness within, from where we can come back out with what we need to face life wholeheartedly.

I have written this book because I know that the only way we can truly thrive in today's world is to reconnect with ourselves, both in our waking hours and while we sleep. Sleep is an act of faith, a deep trust that we can let go of whatever is going on in our lives and sleep deeply with utmost restoration. Sleeping well is about *living* well and I am going to show you how to do this in *Fast Asleep, Wide Awake*.

Mahatma Gandhi said, 'We must become the change we want to see.' In writing this book, I've had to become the change, do the work on myself, go deeper and find my safety so that I can sleep. Although I wonder if this need to go deeper is an evolutionary drive for all of humankind; to force us to come back to ourselves in order to become more aware – to ascend to that next stage of consciousness – and has arisen due to living in this speedy, technological world that constantly urges us 'out there'. I have spent 20-plus years showing people how to become more conscious and self-aware – to wake up and examine their lives and the choices they are making so that they can live deeply and sleep deeply – and even longer learning how to do this myself.

And so, last night I slept without my fan and the explosions and my thoughts were the perfect bedtime story as I drifted effortlessly off to sleep. I slept like a baby (one who sleeps well, that is). I felt safe.

I offer you *Fast Asleep, Wide Awake* with love and deepest gratitude. Writing this book has taken a great deal of hard graft and soul searching – and has called for extraordinary energy and resolve at times – but I always knew that it would be written and felt guided by an unseen but loving and insistent force that kept urging me forwards and encouraged me to 'keep going … keep going'. It is my great privilege to share with you what I have learnt and I do so with an open heart. My prayer is that you read my words with an open and curious mind.

November 2015

Fast Asleep, Wide Awake

Introduction

Thriving Not Surviving

'The ultimate value of life depends upon awareness and the power of contemplation rather than upon mere survival.'

Aristotle

Allow me to share some beliefs that have been very influential in my work and what I am going to share with you in this book. I have arrived at these beliefs as a result of living what I teach for the last 20 years, studying and working with thousands of people. I invite you to take your time and reflect on each belief as each one has the potential to change your relationship with your sleep and energy.

It might be helpful to have a notebook or journal and pen handy to record your thoughts, learning and questions as you read through the book.

Belief #1: Our Body Is Amazing

I am a physiologist and have studied human physiology both for my academic research and out there in the real world. Twenty or more years later, I'm still learning, but our body's capacity to heal and self-regulate never ceases to amaze me.

I know many of the people who turn up at my clinic and in my therapy groups do so because they have lost faith in their body's ability to be at rest and sleep. And if you're feeling shattered due to sleepless nights then it's likely that you too may find it hard to believe. But the simple fact is this: Your body, all 75 or so trillion cells, has an innate intelligence. Each cell contains about 10,000 times as many molecules as the Milky Way has stars.

Our ability to sleep is embedded within our DNA.

Your body knows how to sleep, so what's gone wrong?

A number of factors affect our relationship with sleep and can 'muddy' our sleep engineering, affect our beliefs and attitudes towards sleep, our biochemistry and our brain's ability to regulate our ability to sleep. So you're in the right place because I am going to show you how to clean this all up. I am going to help you to remember how to sleep deeply and effortlessly again.

Belief #2: Sleeping Tablets Are Not the Answer

Your relationship with sleep is unique to you. Your body is designed to create the right type and amount of sleep for you. This means the right amount of dreaming sleep, the right amount of light sleep and the right amount of deep sleep. Your requirements will be different from mine, your partner's or anyone else's. Your biochemical makeup is a unique cocktail of hormones, neuropeptides and neurotransmitters that are designed in a way that is particular to your uniqueness, and is designed to give you perfect sleep. So when you hear about 'the amount of sleep you *should* be getting', this is just a statistical average that fits most of the population – but does it really fit you?

Sleeping pills are a one-size-fits-all sledgehammer approach to treating sleep disorders and so will never be able to give you the type of sleep that you need. Most importantly, they will never be able to give you the type of energy that you need to live your life joyfully and with meaning and purpose. After all, that's why we all want good sleep, isn't it? There's nothing more delicious than having a good night's sleep, but what we're really after is the potential it has to bring us the next day.

Belief #3: Sleep Has an Innate Healing Ability

We are meant to spend roughly a third of our lives sleeping. I still find this statistic astonishing. Why are we designed this way? There must be a reason. There's still so much more to learn about the mysterious process of sleep but what is abundantly clear is that pure sleep has the ability to restore, heal and reorganise those 75 trillion cells. In Sanskrit there is a word *sattvic*, meaning 'pure', and this is the type of sleep that I'll refer to throughout the book.

Sattvic sleep holds the key to healing potential and vibrant energy.

Sattvic sleep is not the junk sleep that many of us get these days (and nights!) – sleep that is muddied by the noise and stimulation of the day – it is clean, pure, deep and restorative.

We need this sleep. Our world is so fast-paced and busy that when we lie down at night we need to recover from the day's demands and allow ourselves to tap into this healing potential.

Belief #4: Insomnia in the 21st Century Has Its Own Particular Significance

Insomnia has been around for a long time and certainly isn't a new phenomenon. There are, however, at least a few factors of modern living that have resulted in sleeping issues becoming much more widespread and, in certain scenarios, the 'norm'.

Speed

Life for most of us is challenging, overwhelming, too busy and way too fast – and this pushes us to do more. This is without even factoring in the real heartbreak stuff that's thrown at us from time to time: illnesses, losing our loved ones, children growing up, parents growing down, relationships falling apart and so on. We cut corners in a futile attempt to get through our inbox or to-do list and regain control, so we eat faster or skip meals, breathe quicker, hug less, laugh less, cry less, love less, feel less – all of this just takes too much time. As Carl Honoré, author of *In Praise of Slow*, says, 'These days, the whole world is time-sick. We all belong to the same cult of speed.'

It's a strange paradox that while we've become obsessed with getting enough sleep we've also become complacent about taking slices off it because, in comparison with everything else, it seems to be a luxury item that we don't need and can't afford. The result is that we prioritise staying awake over resting our bodies and minds, saying, 'I'll get an early night tomorrow … at the weekend … when I'm on holiday … when I retire.' But we can't. Sacrificing sleep night after night leaves us grey and lacklustre and praying for the day when we can take a break. But by the time your backside hits the sunlounger you've fallen prey to some sort of *itis*, or worse. How many of us are walking around saying, 'I'm okay as long as I don't stop. It's only when I stop that I get sick'?

Noise

We seem to have lost the ability to be quiet. Deep restorative sleep is quiet and still. No noise and very little movement. To have this at night we need to touch this depth in our waking hours too, otherwise we become like a hyperactive child – exhausted but unable to settle and sleep. For many, sleep is noisy and fitful. Many of my clients report feeling as though they are neither asleep nor awake. Others say they have to sleep with some noise in the room – a TV or radio. For them, silence feels almost alien and even the sound of their thoughts is threatening. As the 13th-century mystic and theologian Meister Eckhart said, 'There is nothing in the world that resembles God so much as silence.'

So many of us have simply lost the ability to be silent and with silence, and now we are starting to feel the effects. Human beings have always needed to be quiet. Isn't this why we're called human beings not human doings?

The effects of silence on the brain are measurable and studies show that the brain is healthier and less prone to neuro-degeneration with regular daily doses of silence.[1,2] Until fairly recently, quiet time has been innate and not something we've had to engineer. That is, until the world started getting noisier, faster and busier, and we lost our natural and automatic ability to draw our energy and ourselves inwards. No wonder the yoga, meditation and mindfulness movements have become increasingly popular over the last 15 years or so; it is exactly in parallel with the growth of technology that seeks to constantly draw us outwards to connect. We seem to have forgotten that retreating and being silent is not only desirable but also absolutely essential to our being able to replenish and renew our energy before we move to action.

Silence is absolutely essential to being able to sleep deeply and live vibrantly.

Always On, Always Connected

The way we have reacted to technology is causing us some problems, including sleep and energy problems.

Notice that I haven't said that this is due to technology but rather the way we've reacted to it. We are responsible.

This is not a rant against the Internet and other smart devices – I like those things too. Technology was designed to make life easier and in many ways it has, hasn't it? That I can speak to my elderly mother thousands of miles away and see her. That I can sit in my garden studio and communicate with hundreds of people around the world at the same time and make a living from it. That I can reconnect with friends and family I haven't seen for decades and who are now in my life again in a meaningful way. That's good stuff, isn't it?

The problem is that being constantly connected via the Internet has become so pervasive and seductive, so hard to put down, that we just can't switch off and end up running faster, doing more, to keep up – and the impact on our sleep?

Later in this chapter you'll find out what happens to the body and the sleep mechanism when it is constantly bombarded with technology, but for now I'll keep it simple. To sleep deeply we have to live deeply. We have to engage fully with life. If we spend all our time living on the surface of life, responding reactively to demand, how can we ever expect to go deep in our sleep?

Always On, Always Disconnected

We have a whole layer of newly evolved brain, the neocortex, which has the specific purpose of connecting with others, and forming strong bonds and attachments. For relating to others and meeting our basic emotional needs for love, intimacy and trust. However, as Sherry Turkle, the Abby Rockefeller Mauzé Professor of the Social Studies of Science and Technology at the Massachusetts Institute of Technology, wrote in *Alone*

Together, 'Digital connections … may offer the illusion of companionship without the demands of friendship … we'd rather text than talk.' You may be wondering what this has to do with sleep, but it brings me to an important belief that underpins my work.

Belief #5: We Sleep When We Feel Safe

As I mentioned right at the beginning of this book, I have this simple belief that we sleep when we feel safe. Connection – true intimacy, love and trust – is one of the fastest routes to feeling safe. It changes our biochemistry, our brain, our ability to trust, let go, relax and sleep. Technology, with its new ways of relating, has given rise to a kind of biochemical loneliness in which the neocortex drives us to seek out connection, but we're doing it in all the wrong ways. An obvious example is the teenager who reaches for her phone in the early hours to check her social media feed. The dopamine reward from the number of 'likes' offers some short-lived relief from the loneliness but she's left feeling even more wired and unable to sleep.

Every living organism needs to feel safe.

In his book *Feeling Safe*, William Bloom, a leading holistic teacher and author, says, 'Feeling safe is one of the foundations of a normal, happy and fulfilling life. You simply cannot get on with the basic business of living if you feel insecure, frightened, or anxious.'

I extend this to say that to sleep well we need to feel safe. And we need to feel safe regardless of what's going on out there: worries about terrorist attacks, worries about our relationships, our children, elderly parents, our health, our financial and job insecurities, and our overflowing inboxes. Some of this is the real, gritty stuff of life but in order to sleep well – so that we wake with the energy and resilience for whatever needs to be dealt with – we need to get pure, deep sleep.

And herein lies a big problem. Sattvic sleep becomes unattainable when we are running in survival mode because we're operating from the wrong part of our physiology, the part that doesn't allow us to sleep because we need to remain vigilant to fight or flee from the threat (real or perceived), to clear that inbox, meet the demand. Too many of the people who walk through my consulting room door or are sitting in the corporate auditoriums listening to me speak are running in survival mode.

In order to feel safe to sleep we need to break the cycle of surviving.

Belief #6: Sleep Problems Don't Start When You Put Your Head on the Pillow at Night

Every thought, every behaviour, every choice that you make during the day impacts what happens when you place your head on the pillow at night. You carry these energetic vibrations of the day into your sleep and they reverberate within you, keeping you awake or jolting you into sudden heart-thudding wakefulness. Sometimes they slide even deeper into your sleep, creating the stories of nightmares and night terrors, or overwork your muscles so that you wake up drenched and cold with night sweat.

So when I talk to my patients and clients about sleep, it is an invitation to talk about the choices they are making in their waking hours and my next belief.

Belief #7: The Sleep Problem Is Rarely the Real Problem

If you come to see me with a sleep problem I'm going to do my best to help you sleep. During the consultation I'll ask all sorts of questions – you'll learn about some of these questions later – but the simplest and most obvious question I ask is 'Why?' Why is this person not sleeping? I ask this question over and over again (in my mind) during the consultation. Why? Why? Why? Ultimately I want to get to the deepest, innermost source of the problem.

Now I might not, at the time, share the deepest reasons for my client's sleep problem – perhaps they are exhausted and not in a state to hear and/or they know it anyway (although they might not know that they know it). My job – at least initially – is to get them to a point where they're getting some sleep, feeling more energised and robust, *and then* they are ready to look at the true cause of the sleep problem. This is doing what I call 'The Real Work'.

So if you've been struggling for a while, your sleep problem is likely to be a life problem. You might feel it's related to the 10 cups of coffee you are drinking – of course this will stop you sleeping. But *why* are you drinking 10 cups of coffee? *Why* do you need 10 cups of coffee to fund your energy? *Why* is your energy running on such a deficit that you need 10 cups of coffee? This is where The Real Work lies. And this is why superficial sleep hygiene methods and sleeping pills don't and won't work.

A lavender-steeped bath, pleasant as it is, isn't going to truly tackle the source of your sleep problem. Nor is that drug, which is pharmacologically designed to artificially induce a state of sleepiness. Often this is why those with chronic sleep problems end up going from one therapist to another, one book to another, in the hope of finding the solution to their sleeplessness … and never finding it.

The solutions aren't out there. The ultimate solution lies in doing the inner work, The Real Work.

Belief #8: We All Have Access to Amazing, Vibrant Energy

I have arrived at this belief not just as a result of having studied a lot of theory, but I've also worked with a lot of people and, as a result, have learnt a lot about energy. My work has brought me in front of a diverse range of human beings: stressed-out mothers, city employees, children, Premiership footballers, movie and pop stars, prime ministers and their wives, lorry drivers in oil depots, princesses from the Far East. Believe me, I could tell you some stories! Don't forget, along with being a sleep expert, I'm also an energy expert and my work is also about helping people to tap into the amazing, vibrant energy that we all have access to.

Recently I spoke at a conference with over 500 people from a management consultancy firm and asked the question,

'Would you prefer me to show you how to sleep better or how to have amazing energy?' A show of hands indicated that 75 per cent of the people in the room wanted more energy. A week later I gave a presentation to a packed assembly hall of 10-year-olds and asked the same question. This time every single child in the room said they wanted to be shown how to have more energy. Children are wise that way, aren't they?

Why do we give up on our energy? By this I mean settle for less. Why do we think it's impossible to have more energy, to feel extraordinary, to wake up in the morning with a smile, or at least grateful for what lies ahead? Do you think it's possible to feel like this?

A while ago I realised that in helping people overcome their sleep problems something else was happening – something that I hadn't set out to do. Using my sleep formula wasn't only helping them switch off, lie down and sleep, but also tap into more energy. While this might not sound like rocket science – if you sleep well of course you'll have more energy – but the quality of that energy and how it impacted their lives was truly extraordinary.

Was I responsible for this? Were the tools I was sharing bringing about this amazing effect? Well, yes and no. I realised that by helping people with my Fast Asleep, Wide Awake (FAWA) formula they went on to get good sleep but then the sleep started to do its work, which in turn supercharged their energy. Sometimes this happened after just one session. In fact, I very rarely needed to see anyone for more than a few sessions – as long as they were following the FAWA formula, I could take them to a place where their body's innate wisdom then started to do the work.

For example, Simon, a personal trainer, came to see me exhausted and struggling with nightmares. He went on to end a troubled relationship, leave his job and set up a successful fitness business. Or Sarah, a drama student, on the verge of giving up her studies due to sleep problems and fatigue, who has recently been awarded a prestigious award and a fellowship to study in the States.

> **When we are aligned with life, dealing with it head on and not running away, our life force is unlocked and our energy becomes extraordinary.**

Belief #9: This Book Could Change Your Life

If you work through the techniques and exercises progressively as they appear in the book, they will certainly begin to change your life. I have thought hard about using the words 'change your life' because I don't want to offer false promises nor do I wish to sound boastful. But this not-so-humble claim is made on the basis of the feedback I receive from my clients and patients all the time. When I started doing this work it actually took me a while to believe it. But my scientist's brain started to become more convinced as I continued collecting the data.

Belief #10: Your Sleep Problem Might Be a Blessing in Disguise

Ouch! Please don't throw this book at the wall. Trust me, I do know what it feels like to not sleep and feel as if you're the only person in the world awake at 2 a.m. It's horrible. But I am going to show you how to change this and more.

As I've already said, the root cause of any sleep problem is not just about sleep, as there's The Real Work that needs to be done. Invariably, by working with the unique FAWA formula you'll likely to get to the point where you have to do and want to do The Real Work. You'll arrive at the true meaning of your sleep problem and the work then brings about healing in your life (and in turn you sleep better).

If right now you can't even imagine that your sleep 'problem' could be a blessing, can I ask you, just for now, to hold this thought at the back of your mind ... a gentle possibility perhaps? Here are some real-life examples:

- **The woman** who couldn't get to sleep or stay asleep due to supporting her husband through his brain cancer treatment. Doing The Real Work she became aware of her relationship with perfectionism and control. She learnt how to safely feel and express emotions. She learnt how to embrace uncertainty.
- **The university student** who suffered from nightmares and sleepwalking. Doing The Real Work she became aware of her relationship with perfectionism and control. She is learning how to be still and accept herself.
- **The professional athlete** who couldn't sleep before a big game because he kept mentally replaying his failure when he should have been sleeping. Doing The Real Work he became aware of his relationship with perfectionism and control, and how it hindered his ability to perform at his best. He is learning how to deal with failure and visualise success.
- **The 38-year-old city worker** who was exhausted and burnt out from overworking. A near disaster brought him to my

clinic when he fell asleep while standing at the top of the stairs – he was holding his three-month-old daughter at the time. Part of his pattern of overworking was related to his worry that he wasn't good enough so he felt the need to prove himself. Things weren't good at home too and his wife was finding motherhood very difficult. He was carrying the full weight of his wife's problems on his shoulders. Doing The Real Work he became aware of his relationship with perfectionism and control, and is working on self-acceptance and self-esteem. He is learning about boundaries in his personal and professional relationships.

- **The 50-year-old investment banker** who lost his way in life, despite having accumulated significant financial success. He was taking seven different types of medication to quell his anxiety, settle his stomach, control his pre-diabetic condition and cholesterol levels and help him sleep. Doing The Real Work he became aware of how much he had been living in misalignment with his personal values. He is finding meaning and purpose and discovering what true happiness means for him.

- **The HR manager** who couldn't switch off from the demands of her day. For over a year she had been waking in the early hours worrying and finding it hard to get back to sleep. Doing The Real Work she became aware of her relationship with perfectionism and control. She is learning how to manage the boundaries in her relationships at work and home, and how to manage her tendency to over-give at the expense of her own energy. She is building self-esteem and self-acceptance.

- **The accountant** who, after months of sleep deprivation and running in survival mode, was signed off with stress and exhaustion. Doing The Real Work he became aware of his relationship with perfectionism and control. He is finding meaning and purpose.

Are you surprised to see how often 'relationship with perfectionism and control' comes up? Virtually everyone who comes to see me has something going on with his or her relationship with themselves. How they see and speak to themselves. Not feeling good enough. Not loving or even liking themselves. This might have made them successful in many ways – the fear of not being good enough drove them hard, but it came at a cost – they ended up sleepless and exhausted. Later I am going to show you how this absence of self-acceptance and self-love transfers into your sleep, creating a rigidity and inability to accept support. More importantly, I'm going to show you how to fix it.

These 10 beliefs form the philosophy behind my work as a sleep therapist and the FAWA formula. I know you need quick results so here's a summary of how the formula will lead you from surviving to thriving.

The FAWA Formula

Fast Asleep, Wide Awake is in four parts to reflect the tried-and-tested FAWA formula I use with clients and patients whether in my consulting room, in group therapy or in an auditorium. By using the formula you can start to revolution-ise both your sleeping and waking hours, and this is how we roll:

Part I – A Shift in Awareness

Understand what has been going on with your sleep by taking a Personal Reality Check, which consists of the same questions that I would ask you if you were sitting in a consulting room with me and will help you understand your sleep and energy. You may be surprised how simply taking this assessment will bring about a shift in your awareness that will immediately start to influence how you sleep.

Part II – The Energy Clean Up

Apply what I call the '5 Non-negotiables' (5NNs)[3] to recalibrate your nervous system, clean up and free your energy. These five simple but powerful strategies are unique to my work, will very quickly begin to affect your sleep and energy levels – sometimes within just 72 hours of using them – and begin to lay the foundations for the sleep and energy tools to come.

Part III – Fast Asleep: Creating Pure, Deep Sleep

Next you'll be ready for the Pure Sleep Programme to help you refine and deepen the quality of your sleep, and make way for healing and further energy optimisation. The tools here range from small and practical changes that you can make immediately (the Essentials) to the Deeper Tools, which work on the innermost level to bring about even more profound changes, which will also affect your waking hours.

Many of the Deeper Tools are based on Eastern philosophy on energy cultivation and health, and so incorporate yoga, chi kung (*qi gong*), breath exercises, visualisation and mental imagery, affirmations, mantras and more. These techniques work on the factors that influence your sleep at the innermost level. Some of them may be new to you or seem somewhat more esoteric than the more functional tools in Part I, but I simply ask that you try a few of them with an open mind and note how they affect and enhance your energy and wellbeing. What have you got to lose?

Part IV – Wide Awake: Doing The Real Work

In this Energy for Life Programme I share techniques and principles that I have been teaching people, as well as practising myself for a number of years, and as such have been rigorously tried and tested. These exercises and tools will help you to tap in to the physical, emotional, mental and spiritual energy you need to create something more of your life. Be prepared to go deeper with this section.

You might feel tempted to dive straight into the sleep and energy programmes but I ask you to trust the process and go through each of the four stages in turn. As you'll discover in the following chapters, I've developed and fine-tuned the FAWA formula over many years and each step is vital in creating that transformational sleep–energy balance. Therefore, waking up and cleaning up your energy in Parts I and II is a prerequisite to rediscovering the energy you'll need to get the maximum benefit from the programmes that follow in Parts III and IV.

Warning: Side effects from using the four-stage FAWA formula will include finding peace, inner safety and calm amidst the chaos. You may also find that somehow, for some reason, you simply feel less busy although you still get a lot done. Be prepared because you may also begin to experience more happiness and joy.

A New Way of Living and Thriving

I believe that we are in the midst of a very significant time in our evolution – a time when the old ways of being, doing and living are no longer working for us and, if we try to keep doing it the old way, we risk simply burning out. Technology is evolving so fast and it is forcing us to find different ways to go deeper, our DNA cannot keep up and so what we're experiencing is a vital step in our evolution, which is responding out of necessity to enable us to do more than merely survive. All the way down to the cellular level and beyond to the microcellular level, changes are taking place in order to enable us to adapt. Strands of DNA, hitherto thought of as junk, are becoming activated and functional to enable us to adapt to a world that's going faster: to help us think faster, respond faster, live faster. And all due to living in a way that is unnatural to us.

Technology is our greatest drive to evolve – it's a gift.

Nature has given us a way in which we can do this through the magical process of sleep but we need to understand it and learn how to do it in a way that will enable this vital transformation to take place.

The FAWA formula will help you to sleep well but it goes far beyond this. You will learn how to tap into energy that will enable you to start truly living and evolving. I hope that the fact that you're holding my book in your hands means that you are ready to work with me: that you are sick of feeling exhausted, overwhelmed and surviving; that you long to slide effortlessly into pure, deep sleep from which you wake up with the energy to face life.

I've had the immense privilege of being able to help so many people and I continue to do so. I never stop feeling grateful for this, nor do I ever take this for granted. I say thank you every day and several times a day. I am now ready to share what I have learnt.

Chapter 1

Getting Ready to 'Be the Change'

'If you always do what you always did, you will always get what you always got.'

Albert Einstein

Possibly the hardest part of learning to sleep deeply and living vibrantly is acknowledging that something needs to change. You need to change. And change can be painful.

If you know anything about behaviour change you'll already know that it takes a certain amount of time to break a habit and to form a new one – usually about 21 days. Cultivating the right frame of mind by being in a state of receptiveness enables that change to happen more easily and starts to take hold immediately. So before you embark on your mission, you may find the following helpful in preparing your body and mind to becoming the change you seek.

Slow Down and Prepare to Sleep

Slow down as you read. This is not an exercise in speed-reading. Every now and then put the book down and just allow the words to sink in, so that you start to integrate the techniques simply by reading them. This in itself will

21

bring about the softening that is needed for deep sleep to take place.

Prepare to sleep even while you're reading this book. By this I mean, lighten up, drop your shoulders and relax. So many sleep/energy problems are simply due to us trying so hard. To give you an example, when I demonstrate breathing techniques I often observe how – before even starting the exercise – the person will sit bolt upright with an intense look of concentration on their face, jaw clenched, shoulders hunched and, in one case recently, right on the edge of her chair while gripping the seat – as though she was just about to set off on a race!

> **Stop trying so hard. It is this same rigidity, and desperate bid to control, for perfection, to get it right ... that often stops us sleeping in the first place.**

Gentle Discipline

You may find that you'll need to exercise some gentle discipline and give up old ways of being to restore your sleep–energy balance because I'll be asking you to make some changes to your daily routine that may feel uncomfortable or unaccustomed.

Now if you were a teen coming to me with sleep problems, I might have something different to say. I might remove the word 'gentle' from the equation (sometimes I need to be a little tough in order to help bring about changes). I might have to crack the whip to get the electronic devices out of the bedroom in order to help them clean up their act and establish healthy, sleep-conducive routines and habits, as this is what is called for in this situation.

However, I can only ask that you find a balance between applying gentle discipline and strong willpower to make these powerful tools work for you. Are you the perfectionistic, driven, teeth-grinding control freak or a floppy teenager? Forgive the labels but I'm exaggerating for the purpose of illustration. My point is, find your own balance point.

If you decide that a gentler approach is needed, how do you go about this because this stance might be completely alien to you? Well, the first thing is to relax your grip on the goal. I understand that if you haven't been sleeping and you're exhausted, you're desperate to see some results. You might tell yourself, 'I hope this works.' I recommend a subtle shift in mindset in which you become curious rather than goal-focused and you say to yourself, 'I wonder what will happen if I do this?' Do you see the difference? The latter is softer, more open to whatever happens – and that's exactly what is needed to sleep.

Learning to Listen Deeply

For many people listening is a lost skill. In our noisy world we've become so used to living on the surface of life, talking but not really listening, watching but not really seeing, hearing but not really understanding, and because of this we stop feeling too.

When you slow down, you listen and feel what your body is telling you.

When you listen deeply you might start to discern that what you need is to get up and move, rather than have that cup of coffee, or to eat something nourishing, rather than continue sitting there staring at the computer screen. You might spot when your mind is producing a continuous stream of unhelpful thoughts, which are driving even more tension and rigidity into your body. This state usually only becomes apparent when you get into bed at night when you might start to think, 'Where did that come from? I thought I was feeling fine a minute ago.' You might start to notice that, even though you've been consumed and overwhelmed with the worries of your life, there are also a few (and actually maybe more than a few) gifts that you'd stopped noticing – that you're taking for granted and have stopped seeing.

I realised a long time ago that one of the most important aspects of my job is really helping people to listen and notice deeply – to become more conscious. I emphasise the word 'deeply' because, if we can get to a place of deep listening and noticing, then a kind of magic starts to happen and we start making the right, the most intelligent, choices. I don't mean exam-passing, credential-attaining intelligence but a more inward-focused body-mind intelligence that starts to steer us in the best possible direction – deeper sleep, more energy and better life choices.

Breathe Deeply

So right now I invite you to wake up your ability to listen deeply. This is the first, vital step to becoming more conscious.

1. Sit comfortably. Place both feet firmly on the floor. Straighten up and breathe deeply into your belly and exhale long and slow.
2. Imagine sending that exhalation out through the lower half of your body and out through your feet. Breathe back in feeling your belly expand outwards.
3. Repeat the first two steps, but this time with your eyes closed. And now feel into your body. Is there any tightness or any rigidity? Feel your body ... listen to it ... what does it want? What is it telling you?

I was surprised when I did this simple breathing exercise while writing these words. I took my hands off the keyboard and followed my own instructions. I found myself leaning back a little and stretching the front of my chest, and as I did so I heard a little click as tension was released from my breastbone. (I didn't even know that was there.) I opened my arms, as if stretching my wings, and felt a blissful stretch in my shoulders and upper back. (I didn't even know my shoulders and back were tense.) I found myself releasing a sigh, 'AAAAHHH.' Now that I've straightened up and opened my eyes, I find I can breathe slightly more deeply. And I'm feeling somewhat more focused and relaxed at the same time.

Maintain a Relaxed State of Focus

Keep doing this as you read. Keep working on the art of listening deeply and noticing. You will find that you start receiving more and more 'data' from your intelligent body. And you'll begin to find that you are more able to understand exactly what this data is guiding you to do.

> Beware of resistance and protest – you may read something and think, 'This is something I've never done and could never do.' Strangely, this might be the very thing that you do need to do.

Imagine yourself in a vision of what you want to create – see yourself getting into bed and melting gratefully, without resistance, into a deep, nourishing sleep. See yourself waking in the morning, again with gratitude for the sleep you've had. See yourself moving with energy to meet your day with open heart and mind.

Chapter 2

Discovering the FAWA Formula

'All life is an experiment. The more experiments you make the better.'

Ralph Waldo Emerson

The FAWA formula isn't something I learnt from a textbook or studied at university. Sure, I've studied for degrees and read a lot of books, but what I'm going to share in the following chapters comes from an inside-out approach that brings together several strands: academic studies, professional research and observations from my work. Much of my work is intuitive, perhaps because I have also been my own patient, and often I have found myself knowing something and then, with great relief, and sometimes years later, find the scientific evidence and data to validate what I have always known.

However, it was a lecture on homeostasis – maintaining internal balance and constancy – that finally woke me up to my life's work. At the time I wasn't quite sure why this particular lecture was worth listening to, but later, as I struggled to maintain a sense of balance in my own life, it all became clear.

At the time I was studying for a Doctorate in Physiology but, I guess like many students, I struggled to get out of bed in the morning and was more intent on having a good time.

Even back then, I knew it was possible to sleep with your eyes open.

This time, I didn't fall asleep. Instead I was entranced by the lecturer's words as he spoke about how every biological process in the body – temperature, appetite, cellular fluid balance, breathing, heartbeat and the sleep–wake cycle – oscillates around a set point, following a sinusoidal up and down rhythm, as shown in Figure 1 below.

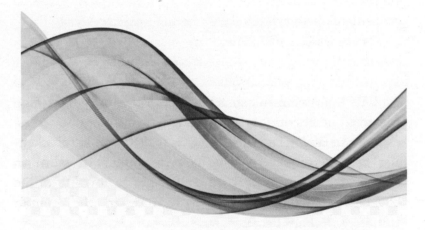

Figure 1: *The natural rhythm of physiological processes*

The more I studied (and paid attention), the more I became fascinated by how intricately and intelligently the body works to create balance, even in rapidly changing external conditions.

A few years down the line, I found myself in a City of London health-screening clinic measuring the physiology and wellbeing of lawyers, bankers and other corporate employees, and this was when things started to change for me and the FAWA formula was born.

Righting the Balance

I loved helping people to understand what was going on with their sleep patterns and energy levels, showing them how the world was impacting them and what they could do to stay in balance, offering reassurance and hope. I was particularly interested to notice that what I measured in the lab didn't quite match what l learnt in my academic training; there was a mismatch between the theory and the practice.

My measurements seemed to indicate that people attending the clinic were overusing their fight-or-flight system or sympathetic nervous system (SNS). In other words, living as though they were in perpetual survival mode. Breathing patterns and respiratory measures, electrocardiogram traces, blood tests and even body fat levels (called 'trunkal thickening' to diplomatically describe a thickening waistline in response to stress) all provided data about how life in the speedy City was creating imbalance in the human physiology.

This was at a time when technology was increasing at an exponential rate as the Internet, mobile phones and email had just exploded on to the scene. Everything and everyone was accelerating. Our physiology was being stretched to its limits and I was seeing this in real time in the measurements I was taking in my lab.

Helping my clients to learn to keep up, adapt, and stay healthy and sane while going at this pace, I was fascinated to measure the changes in their physiological data when they came back to see me three months later. When they took my advice and used the FAWA formula, I saw how it made a measurable difference – even though they were just making relatively small changes. A grateful CEO asked me to develop a programme for his team that could be delivered in their corporate offices to teach his staff what he had learnt in clinic. I called this workshop 'Managing the Pace' and within a year I had feedback from over 1,000 employees who had attended it.

It seems to be the small changes that make all the difference to our lives.

Since then I have shared the same formula in corporate auditoriums speaking to hundreds of people hungry for solutions to their sleep problems and exhaustion. As technology advanced, I found myself working virtually and globally across time zones and continents, sometimes sitting in my office at home and helping people around the world to get better sleep and to break out of the fatigue cycle.

Among my 'well' clients I also worked in a psychiatric clinic, helping those suffering with a host of mental illnesses including anxiety, depression, addictions, eating disorders, work-related stress and burnout, and my sleep and energy programmes soon became the most rewarding area of my work. Not only because I was helping people to find a way out of the most seemingly desperate of circumstances but also, perhaps, because I had once been a patient at that very same clinic years ago.

Waking Up

The seed of the FAWA formula comes from my personal journey.

The truth is that even while doing well academically and professionally, my personal life was shambolic. I was racked with fear and drove myself hard, all the time feeling that I really wasn't good enough and worrying that I'd be found out. Sleep was a big issue and I was plagued by insomnia, lying in bed at night tortured by my own thoughts. In fact, it was this crazy sleep pattern that inspired the title of my first book, *Tired But Wired*.

It wasn't that I didn't have energy – but it was the wrong kind of energy: buzzing, hyper, anxious and restless, on edge and running in survival mode. At university, my friends thought I was the life and soul of the party, not realising that often my 'gaiety' was a big act, masking fear and insecurity, that would later plummet into depression and exhaustion when on my own.

I had a sense that things weren't right but felt powerless to change anything. Why was I this way? My childhood hadn't been easy or stable at the best of times, so perhaps this was partly responsible for my restlessness and inability to settle to sleep. I know it caused my mother great heartache – she even took me to a doctor when I was six months old because I wouldn't sleep. But my earliest memories are of being a bit odd, not quite fitting in, sensing so much but not being able to articulate how I was feeling – and fear, which seemed to pervade my life.

A life-changing moment came in 1998 when, in a state of despair, I travelled to Australia for six months. I didn't really have a plan but knew I had to get away from everything – a clinical label that I didn't believe, a marriage that wasn't working, therapy that didn't seem to be getting me anywhere, medication that wasn't making any difference. Here everything slowed down and my view of life changed. Suddenly everything became very clear to me. I could see that the choices I'd been making had kept me stuck and created *dis*-ease in my mind and body. In this brief moment I also found something within me – a refuge and stillness – and from this place I was able to see life differently and make profoundly different choices. I can only describe this as coming home, or touching God. Whatever it was, I surrendered and let go, and from that moment my life changed.

Deepening the Learning

After this awakening, I began to learn about balance and life, but in a different way to the way I'd been taught in conventional academia. What I'd been feeling and sensing suddenly began to make sense, and as if by magic, as I learnt more, opportunities to teach others from my experiences started turning up.

The most significant shift was in my relationship with fear – which had been blocking my happiness, my energy and life force, and stopping me from sleeping – and as I learnt how to sleep deeply and balance my energy, so my work with others deepened and flourished. I was so excited about these changes in my life and how I was feeling that I was hungry to learn more. I devoured books on healing and Eastern philosophy. I read about energy medicine and physics (a favourite subject at school), and the work of medical practitioners and doctors such as Dr Deepak Chopra and Dr Lissa Rankin who had both turned to holistic practices to bring about healing in their own lives and their patients. I attended workshops and seminars and experimented with different types of yoga and meditation. As I learnt I continued to heal myself and my own life, I took this learning into my work and delighted in finding new ways of bringing exhausted, sleep-deprived cynics (those corporate auditoriums) along with my thinking.

When I started delving deeper into the Eastern sciences, I began to get very excited by what I was learning about energy (probably because of my own personal challenges to manage my own energy). Western science and physics had taught me that energy was 'the physical capacity to do work' but in the ancient texts I started to learn more about life force energy.

Our life force, our energy, sits at the centre of our lives, enabling us to realise our potential, to achieve, to do whatever we need to do to get through the day and more, to be well and healthy and free of disease. When this energy is vibrant, it enables us to be the best that we can be. When we're wide awake and filled with this life force, living just seems so much easier. We can cope with life's challenges and demands. We make better decisions and more informed choices, acknowledge what is possible, sort the wheat from the chaff and get through our days feeling bright and in control.

Living with extraordinary energy fuels every day with more happiness and joy.

We can now measure this energy, as the Russian-born physicist Dr Konstantin Korotkov – a pioneer in the field of human energy measurement – has developed highly innovative technology for measuring the life force of all living organisms, including plants. His Gas Discharge Visualisation (GDV) technology has identified that all living things have an energy field that is measurable and is affected by their environment, external forces and influences.[4] GDV technology is now being used in Russia for medical diagnostics and increasing numbers of clinicians are using it in everyday practice. Now it is also being used in more than 40 countries for research and for the analysis of human energy fields. What this tells me, and I hope it makes you excited too, is this:

Our life force not only exists but we can supercharge it by applying the *Fast Asleep, Wide Awake* formula.

How the FAWA Formula Works

Starting in 2010, and looking over the data from thousands of clients, I began to see a clear pattern of how my clients and patients were overcoming their sleep problems to finding the energy to truly engage with life. I noticed that whether I was working face to face in my consulting room or with hundreds of people in an auditorium, healing seemed to follow the same five-step formula:

Step 1: Shifting Awareness

The first step of the formula is focused on helping you understand what is going on with your sleep and your energy. This stage of my work often brings about a shift in awareness, which is crucial in being able to take responsibility and make different choices. In *Tired But Wired* I describe this as the ARC of transformation:

- awareness
- responsibility
- choices

So an important part of this process is digging deep within so that you can understand why things have become a certain way and, importantly, what you need to do about it, as well as undertaking a personal reality check. You'll also find how your beliefs can play a significant role in how you sleep. The questions I invite you to reflect on in your Personal Reality Check (*see Chapter 5*) are the same ones I would ask you if you were sitting with me in a consulting room at my clinic.

Step 2: Cleaning Up Your Energy

This next step is where my expertise as a physiologist really comes into play, and I cannot overemphasise the importance of this stage of the programme.

Often very soon after meeting my client/patient, I can make an intuitive assumption of how their nervous system is running – whether it's in SAFETY or SURVIVAL mode. The questions I then ask – the ones you will reflect on in your Personal Reality Check – will validate this assumption.

Next I recommend five strategies, the 5 Non-negotiables (5NNs), to be implemented for at least the next 21 days. These five small strategies change the tuning of the nervous system and shift it from SURVIVAL mode to SAFETY mode. Once this vital recalibration has taken place the other sleep and energy tools can be applied to even more powerful effect. Conversely, these tools are totally ineffective if you're running in SURVIVAL mode.

Another important aspect of using the 5NNs is that when you're in a state of exhaustion you need some quick wins. You need to experience some positive changes – improved sleep and energy – to keep you moving forwards and to prepare you for the deeper work to come, and this is exactly what this step of the FAWA formula is designed to do.

The 5NNs are simple and doable – important if you're exhausted and running on empty.

Soon you will learn exactly how to apply these 5NNs, but if you're feeling intrigued they are to do with:

- How and what you eat and drink.
- What you do before your head hits the pillow.
- Your relationship with information and technology.

Step 3: Refining Sleep Quality and Depth

Once the 5NNs have been applied, your body and nervous system are in a much more responsive state and you'll be ready to work with the Pure Sleep Programme. The tools in this section range from simple, commonsense and practical

Essentials to weird and wonderful Deeper Tools, incorporating techniques that I've learnt from Eastern philosophy and Traditional Chinese Medicine (TCM). These techniques are based on sciences that have been around for thousands of years and they really work – I have seen this even with clients who've come to me with a lifelong history of sleep problems that has run in the family for generations. (Don't forget, my original training is as a Western scientist and I am constantly looking for data to support my findings.)

These tools work by activating the branch of the nervous system that enables you to sleep. Your sleep will start to be more refined and deeper. You may still experience occasional sleep difficulties but they will feel less catastrophic because your energy levels will have lifted due to the energy clean-up in Step 2. You will notice that, as you worry less about not sleeping, this in itself – the absence of worry – leads to better sleep. It makes sense, doesn't it?

To sleep beautifully you almost need to not care about how you sleep.

Step 4: Doing The Real Work and Tapping into Vibrant Energy

At this point, you'll be ready for me to share a very special programme with you. The Energy for Life Programme will support you in doing The Real Work. With these tools you can explore happiness and meaning along with dealing with relationships, uncertainty and fears.

Years ago my work with sleep took a strange turn and I, a physiologist and sleep expert, found myself on stages in packed-out auditoriums talking about such things. But why? It's quite simple really – in my quest to solve people's sleep problems (and my own) I ended up talking about the very things that were stopping people from sleeping and draining their energy levels – absence of happiness and purpose, conflict in relationships, fear and uncertainty, and so on. Most significantly, in all of the tools I shared I seemed to be showing people how to reconnect with a part of themselves that had been missing or neglected. And what is this part? Well, you might want to call it spirit or even soul or God.

Earlier I described how my awakening felt like I was coming back to a very familiar place – coming home. However you choose to label it, when you reconnect with this part of yourself it will lead you back to peace, safety, better sleep and vibrant energy.

I hasten to add that the contents of the Energy for Life Programme are not original to me but rather they come from an ancient wisdom that has become all the more relevant in this crucial stage of our history when technology has brought with it a type of magic which – although wonderful in so many ways – ever seeks to draw us out of ourselves and away from our spirit and true source of safety. So my humble intention in sharing this toolkit is to remind you (because for some of you there will be no big surprises here), in practical and concrete ways, how to reconnect with your innermost self and spirit, so that you can sleep deeply and awaken with the vibrant energy needed to live a meaningful life.

My even deeper intention is that you will make these tools and practices part of your everyday life and that you will share them with your children, as it is perhaps the younger generation who are especially in need, at present, of reconnection with soul and spirit.

So here you have it – the unique Fast Asleep, Wide Awake formula. In the following chapters you'll begin to understand some of the most important principles behind why you might be exhausted and not sleeping. Know that as you read and engage with my words the healing process has already begun.

Part I
Shifting Awareness

'I think the key to transforming your life is to be
aware of who you are.'

Dr Deepak Chopra

Chapter 3

Understanding the Sleep–Energy Balance

'Nothing in life is to be feared, it is only to be understood.'

Marie Curie

I deliberated hard before adding this section on sleep because you will find that there is some theory to absorb and it's definitely not my aim to blind (or bore) you with science – particularly if you're feeling tired. However, an important part of this work is about making better choices. I know that it is with this clarity that a shift in awareness is created that is vital for change to occur.

So please don't be tempted to skip this chapter as you will learn a great deal here. Of course, I see some pretty extreme cases at my clinic, notably parasomnia – nightmares, night terrors, sleepwalking and talking – but even these can be overcome when you understand exactly what is going on and how, by making small changes, these distressing symptoms can be avoided.

Surviving or Thriving

If you're out of balance and not sleeping, you might be running on the wrong type of energy. It's a chicken-and-egg situation because the wrong type of energy affects our ability to sleep, and not sleeping sends us further into the wrong type of energy. But what do I mean by 'the wrong type of energy'?

So far I have been using two labels, which I will continue to use throughout this book – SAFETY and SURVIVAL. I use them to describe the two energy modes or systems that human beings have evolved to enable us to live.

The SURVIVAL energy system is the 'fight or flight' system, discovered by the scientist Walter Cannon in the 1920s. We use this in crisis and when we're under threat from predators, when there are inadequate food supplies, harsh climatic conditions or poor shelter. This system resides in a primitive part of the brain called the limbic system within the amygdala. Although, for most of us, the nature of threat has changed in today's world, we still use this survival system when we perceive that we're under threat. In SURVIVAL mode we run on adrenalised fear-driven energy and we don't sleep, as it's not conducive to surviving.

In the SAFETY energy system we produce the hormones of wellbeing – you'll learn more about these shortly and I'll actually show you how to produce them in Part IV. The body's resources are used for healing, repair, growth and development. In SAFETY mode, life feels harmonious and we sleep.

SAFETY SYSTEM	SURVIVAL SYSTEM
Wellbeing	Fight/flight
Healing	Fearful
Growth and repair	Anxious
Sleep	Distrustful
	Vigilant

Table 1: *The SAFETY and SURVIVAL systems*

The autonomic nervous system (ANS) determines which of these energy systems is more active. It runs the length of the body and is divided into two branches:

The parasympathetic nervous system (PNS), the SAFETY branch of the nervous system – which runs the body when we are in rest, repair, healing and sleep mode – is vital for maintaining everyday functions from the integrity of cell functioning to the heartbeat and how we breathe and sleep. The PNS ticks over quietly, keeping us well via the activity of the vagus nerve, which runs from the diaphragm and abdomen through to the brainstem. This important nerve maintains your health, enabling healing and repair. It is also connected to the circadian timer, the sleep control centre in the pineal gland in the brain. Keep it in mind because many of the tools I'm going to share with you are focused on activating it.

The sympathetic nervous system (SNS), the SURVIVAL branch, kicks in when we're in fight-or-flight mode, when we feel stressed or anxious. We need this stress-hormone-producing part of the nervous system to help us perceive and react to threat. The body is flooded with adrenaline, noradrenaline and cortisol, and we are ready to fight or flee. The SNS was essential to our early hunter-gatherer ancestors, as we faced harsh and unsafe conditions, food was scarce and we had to face off wild animals or tribes. But in modern times the SNS is more likely to be activated by a difficult phone call or meeting, the kids playing up in the car or a stressful journey to work and an overflowing inbox.

When we're in balance these two branches of the nervous system operate in harmony throughout the day, swinging back and forth like a pendulum, affecting our energy levels, the rest–activity balance, our motivation and drive, how we feel – hungry, thirsty, hot or cold, sleepy or focused – and these rhythms produce the fluctuations in our mood and energy throughout the day, the hum of our energy. The pendulum swings back and forth between the SNS and PNS roughly on a 90-minute cycle called the ultradian cycle.[5] We will return to this shortly when we look at how the ultradian cycle plays out while you sleep.

The reality is that a healthy balance can be elusive with our 21st-century lifestyle forcing us to go faster and faster. Many people end up in a state of constant hyperactivity in which the SNS is always in go mode – so-called 'sympathetic overdrive' – and the PNS shuts down. We begin to run on adrenaline, noradrenaline and cortisol, we feel as if we can't stop, life feels chaotic and over-busy, and we get sick as soon as we stop (a classic sign of sympathetic overdrive). And of course we can't sleep. Or if we do, sleep is noisy, jagged and exhausting.

The Effect of Survival Mode on Our Energy

Survival energy is adrenalised, edgy, anxious, restless, impatient, threatened, fearful, hyper-vigilant at one extreme and then plummeting into exhausted, apathetic, hopeless giving up. With my patients I see greater extremes of manic and psychotic, which fall into the trough of depressed and suicidal. These are the roots of bipolar disorder.

Conversely, when we are running on sustainable energy, on the higher end of the scale, we feel vibrant, joyful, passionate, exhilarated and positively challenged. In its lower state, sustainable energy feels pleasantly tired, mellow and chilled out. Sustainable energy is about feeling safe and in this state we run on the safety hormones of love and wellbeing – serotonin and oxytocin. We produce the hormone melatonin – and so can sleep. We need all of these energy states and feelings but we don't want to be stuck in SURVIVAL mode. Many people have become so used to existing in this way – they have habituated to this type of energy – and they can't imagine it being any other way.

SURVIVAL ENERGY	SUSTAINABLE ENERGY
High Negative	**High Positive**
Angry	Invigorated
Fearful	Confident
Defensive	Challenged
Resentful	Joyful
	Connected
Low Negative	**Low Positive**
Depressed	Relaxed
Exhausted	Mellow
Burnt Out	Peaceful
Hopeless	Tranquil
Defeated	Serene

Table 2: *Survival and sustainable energy*

Looking at Table 2 above, ask yourself the following questions and take a note of your answers:

- Where do you feel your energy lies at the moment?
- How has it been recently?
- Are you feeling safe or are you running in survival?

Now let's look at what happens when you sleep – pure sleep.

Pure Sleep

This is relevant for you even if you consider yourself to be a 'good sleeper'. Some people define being a good sleeper as the ability to fall asleep and stay asleep easily, and they might say, 'I haven't got a problem sleeping but I just can't get out of bed.' Remember, there is a vital distinction between sleeping and pure sleep – the ultimately restorative and rejuvenating sleep with just the right amount of dream process and the right amount of deep, dreamless sleep in which you do nothing other than be. Such sleep has an innate organising power: it sorts out our emotional world, clears and tidies our mental filing cabinets, and heals and rebalances the body. From such sleep you wake feeling and looking deeply refreshed, and ready to face life with open arms.

The Benefits of Pure Sleep

According to well-validated Western scientific studies there are three main reasons why we spend so much of our lives sleeping.[6]

Restore
To help us recover from the demands of being awake.

Protect and Clean Up the Brain (the Cortex)
During our waking hours mental activity stimulates the production of natural chemical messengers in the brain called 'excitatory transmitters'. These transmitters can become toxic to the brain. Scientists at the University of Rochester Medical Center have recently discovered a system that drains waste products from the brain as we sleep. Cerebrospinal fluid, a clear liquid surrounding the brain and spinal cord, moves through the brain along a series of channels that surround the blood vessels. The brain's glial cells manage the system and so the researchers called it the 'glymphatic system'. It is thought that it is particularly active during deep sleep and helps to remove a toxic protein called beta-amyloid from brain tissue. This protein is renowned for accumulating in the brains of patients with Alzheimer's disease.[7]

Learning and Memory Consolidation
Sleeping sorts out our mental filing cabinets so we wake up feeling mentally sharp and clear. I'm going to tell you more about this vital function later because for some people it is the reason why they wake up exhausted, feeling as if they've been thinking all night or even oversleeping in a vain attempt to recoup energy.

Many others and I also believe that sleep serves a couple more vital roles. These roles are perhaps not as well validated by Western science but have been identified and explored by older sciences such as Indian Ayurveda (medicine) and Traditional Chinese Medicine (TCM) for thousands of years.

Restore Life Force Energy

Time and again my work has shown how people are able to regain some special part of themselves when they start sleeping well. For example, the actress/singer who was too exhausted and depressed to get out of bed who started singing again and signed a record deal within six months; or the stressed mother who sets up her own company. It's more than just having a good night's sleep and more energy, it's a rekindling of passion, inspiration and courage.

Pure sleep is an awakening of spiritual energy.

Self-healing

The healing benefits of sleep are related to all of the above functions but I feel they deserve highlighting. What happens when you sleep on a problem and wake up feeling better? Or when you go to bed with aches and pains and wake up with no pain at all? Or if you cut yourself and wake up and the wound has virtually disappeared? The body is constantly renewing itself. Up to 75 trillion cells repairing, regenerating and rebalancing. This process is fast-tracked when you sleep.

The Journey Through the Night

There's a kind of magic that takes place when you sleep. Sleep is not one constant state, but rather a progression through various states with extremely unique characteristics.

Earlier I mentioned the 90-minute ultradian cycle, describing it as setting the hum of your energy. This cycle continues throughout the night as we sleep in 90-minute cycles.

Disruption of these cycles when we cross time zones causes sleep disruption and jetlag. The hormones, neurotransmitters and the circadian timer in the pineal gland beautifully orchestrate all this activity.

This important gland in the brain's hypothalamus is also known in Eastern medicine as 'the third eye', and it is sensitive to the daily cycle of light and dark. So when the light level entering our eyes and hitting the light-sensitive retina at the back of the eye drops below 200 lux, this switches on the circadian timer and stimulates the production of the all-important sleep hormone melatonin. The healing PNS becomes more active and the sleep cycle is switched on. The awake cycle is stimulated as light levels increase via a group of cells, also located in the hypothalamus, called the Suprachiasmatic nucleus (SCN). The SCN suppresses the production of melatonin and signals the body that it's time to wake up. The active 'doing' SNS switches on, body temperature increases and hormones such as cortisol are produced to get us going. Every organ system in the body receives a signal to up-regulate (get active) or down-regulate (slow down) and in this way our physiology is kept in an optimal state of balance and fine-tuning.

Western sleep science is relatively young and we are still learning more. Spending a night in a sleep clinic generates polysomnograph recordings, which are measurements of brain wave activity during sleep. The patient is wired up to monitoring equipment with electrodes and an EEG (electroencephalogram tracing of the bioelectric activity of the brain) is produced, which informs the sleep clinician about the person's sleep patterns and potential disorders. In 1937 Alfred Lee Loomis, an American also known for significant work in developing radar, first described the stages of sleep. Loomis and his team used EEG recordings to identify five different levels of sleep.[8] In 1953, another team of scientists discovered that REM (rapid eye movement) sleep was a distinct state, leading to a rethinking of the way sleep was designed and giving us the model we use today.[9]

The Five Stages of Sleep

So let's look at each sleep stage in turn as it may help you to get a sense of why our sleep (and energy levels) may be less than ideal.

In total, there are five stages of sleep that can be easily distinguished from each other: two are light sleep, the following two are slow-wave or deep sleep and the fifth is a short 15-minute burst of REM sleep. Sleep can also be divided into two entirely different states:

1. REM (rapid eye movement) sleep
2. non-REM (nREM) sleep

Additionally, non-REM is subdivided into four sub-stages, which are distinguishable by levels of brain-wave activity. The sleep science community has more recently combined non-REM stages 3 and 4 into one stage (stage 3).

A typical night's sleep consists of about 75 per cent non-REM and 25 per cent REM sleep. The 90-minute cycle repeats throughout the night, each time taking us through the five layers from light to deep sleep and REM sleep. Although I keep emphasising the importance of deep sleep, each of these layers is vital and we have to go through them all while we sleep.

Non-REM Sleep

The first four phases of sleep are non-REM sleep and during these phases, unlike REM sleep, we can move around. Neck and jaw movements are the most common movements. If you suffer from teeth grinding (bruxism) or restless legs syndrome (RLS) both of these are more likely to be evident in the first two stages.

Fully Alert and Awake

In this stage of full consciousness, an EEG brain trace would show a predominance of beta-wave activity. This, of course, is where we spend most of our waking hours. This is the thinking, information processing and mentally alert mode, apparently processing 30,000–50,000 thoughts per day. This is the most overworked layer of our consciousness and one that has started to intrude into our sleep, as you will now see.

Stages 1 and 2 – Light Sleep

These are the first phases of sleep that we enter from being fully awake and alert and here there is predominantly alpha wave activity. Sleep is light and lasts a few minutes, and can be easily interrupted by a gentle nudge, snoring or even – very commonly – thoughts. These sleep phases are initiated when your melatonin levels and sleep debt (level of sleepiness built up throughout the day) are at their highest and, while it could be the easiest phase to slide into, it must be entered with care.

By this I mean falling asleep on the sofa in front of the TV in the evening can sabotage your efforts to subsequently enter the next stages of sleep, as you can deplete your melatonin levels and then find you just can't get to sleep. This problem is exacerbated if you then sneak a look at your emails or social media notifications, as blue light is a potent suppressor of melatonin.

These first two phases of light sleep are the essential warm-up and preparation for deep sleep. We let go of the tension and accumulated stress of the day. Have you ever fallen asleep and then woken with a jerk and a sensation of falling? This is called a hypnagogic jerk and it's most likely to happen in the early stages of falling asleep and releasing the tension of the day. A bit like when you switch your car engine off after a long drive and the engine makes ticking noises as it cools down. It is when we've released the tension of the day that we're 'allowed' access to the deepest levels of rest that are available in deep sleep.

Stages 3–4 – Deep Sleep

In deep, dreamless, non-REM sleep, delta wave activity predominates and it is likely that our deepest restoration comes from this stage. There is virtually no dreaming or body movement. As with REM sleep, these deep sleep phases vary in duration throughout the night. The first 90-minute cycle of sleep tends to be made up mostly of deep sleep with just 7–10 minutes of REM sleep. I'd like you to pause for a moment and reflect on this:

The earliest part of your sleep houses your longest and deepest phases of deep sleep.

Many people are missing out on this stage of sleep because they delay going to bed. Often it's because we worry we have too much to do, emails and social media to check, 'I need some me time,' or 'I just want to watch the next episode in the box set.' When you start cleaning up your sleep and energy in Part I, you will see how relevant this early sleep really is to feeling rested and energetic.

Recently, scientists have been able to demonstrate, using sophisticated polysomnography, that in our modern, busy world 'beta spikes' are disrupting our deep delta sleep. In other words, they can measure that even when the person is in deep sleep there is some beta wave activity within the delta waves – similar to being in a completely dark room and a bright light being constantly switched on and off.[10] My belief is that these sleep 'intrusions' are being caused by over-exposure to technology.

These two factors – delayed sleep and beta intrusions – suggest that many people aren't sleep deprived as such but are deep sleep deprived; hence their exhaustion and perception that they're not getting enough sleep.

Stage 5 – Rapid Eye Movement (REM) Sleep

The rapid eye movements from which REM sleep takes its name are the result of the brain trying to scan the events in the dream world. In other words, if you look left and right in your dream, then your eyes will follow the dream and move left and right under your eyelids. This is known as the scanning hypothesis. The body goes into a state of paralysis here, otherwise you might follow the movement of your eyes and start acting out your dreams.

The REM stages vary in duration throughout the night. The first REM stage in the earliest part of the night is typically the shortest at around 7–10 minutes, but as sleep progresses through the night the REM stages become longer – around 45 minutes. While deep sleep is vital, so is REM sleep. In laboratory studies, rats who usually live for two or three years, if deprived of REM sleep live only three weeks on average.[11] REM sleep begins with signals from an area at the base of the brain called the pons. These signals travel to the thalamus in the brain, which relays them to the cerebral cortex – the outer layer of the brain that is responsible for learning, thinking and organising information. The pons also sends signals that shut off neurons in the spinal cord, causing temporary paralysis of the limb muscles.

REM sleep stimulates the brain regions used in learning. This may be important for normal brain development during infancy, which would explain why babies spend much more time in REM sleep than adults. One study found that REM sleep affects learning of certain mental skills. People taught a skill and then deprived of non-REM sleep could recall what they had learned after sleeping, while people deprived of REM sleep could not.[12]

Your brain is in a highly active stage during REM sleep as vital work is being carried out to file and consolidate the information from the day. In today's information-filled world we really rely on this phase to pack away the information of the day in the brain's working memory so that we wake up feeling mentally sharp and clear.

Sometimes we even fall into this trance-like state – called a hypnagogic trance – during the day. You might have noticed this when, for example, you've been staring at a screen for too long, bombarding the brain with information. By slipping into a trance-like state the brain cleverly seeks a way of going 'offline', in order to empty our mental filing cabinets so that we can come back to the task in hand with renewed focus. Children often do this when they've been concentrating hard – a glazed-over state which signals that the brain is trying to process and consolidate information. Other times you might feel like this when you're driving (which could be dangerous and is the reason why you need to take regular pit stops on long journeys), sitting in meetings (go on, admit it!), or even while watching TV or reading a book. This is an open-eyed trance state in which we are neither awake nor asleep but the brain is vitally seeking to clean up and clear up information.

Herein lies another reason why you might not be getting enough deep sleep. If you've spent a great deal of your day looking at screens and information, and especially before you go to bed, there will be a greater need for sorting and filing. Simply, you'll need more REM sleep. I'm sure you've had nights where it feels as if you haven't slept at all because of the maddening level of mental activity. This is called 'paradoxical insomnia' in which it feels as if you haven't slept at all (and a sleep study in a laboratory would show that you have slept) but it feels as if you haven't.

So I want to emphasise that there are at least three factors compromising our deep sleep:

1. delaying the first sleep phase
2. beta intrusions
3. increased need for REM sleep

Much of this evidence points to how we're using technology and you can see why if we want to improve our sleep and energy levels we have to master our relationship with technology.

Dreaming Sleep

It appears that we do most of our dreaming during REM sleep, and, as our longest period of REM is in the early hours, we do some serious dreaming before we wake up feeling that we have 'spent the whole night dreaming'. We typically spend more than 2 hours each night dreaming and even if you can't remember your dreams you're still dreaming. Dreaming is a fascinating subject, isn't it? Scientists are learning more about how and why we dream. Sigmund Freud, who greatly influenced the field of psychology, believed dreaming was a 'safety valve' for unconscious desires. Only after 1953, when researchers first described REM in sleeping infants, did scientists begin to carefully study sleep and dreaming. They soon realised that the strange, illogical experiences we call dreams almost always occur during REM sleep. While most mammals and birds show signs of REM sleep, reptiles and other cold-blooded animals do not.

Why are our dreams so outlandish and dramatic? Some scientists believe dreams are the cortex's attempt to find meaning in the random signals that it receives during REM sleep. The cortex is the part of the brain that interprets and organises information from our environment when we're awake. It may be that, given random signals from the pons during REM sleep, the cortex tries to interpret these signals as well, creating a story out of fragmented brain activity. I believe that when we sleep we return to a child-like vulnerable state in which our unconscious mind is allowed free rein and becomes almost like an out-of-control computer with unlimited creative capacity. Sometimes this creativity can give rise to such dreams that we wake up alarmed and distressed or even inspired and entertained.

REM Sleep Disorder

In REM sleep disorder the person, distressingly, starts to physically follow their dreams. I have worked with many people who have done bizarre and strange things at night. In fact, as a child I used to sleep walk and talk on a regular basis, as did my father. Recently I worked with an actress who would get up at night and do the most amazing nail art sketches. Another client, a highly intelligent philosophy and drama student, would get up during the night and walk down to the lake in her university campus. Obviously this could have been dangerous and her friends organised a system for keeping an eye on her during the night so that she didn't come to any harm. Another client, Ed, jumped out of his second-storey bedroom window while asleep.

People who have a tendency to act out their dreams are usually creative types who have to learn to manage their creative process, otherwise it literally takes them over at night.

Important Note

I don't refer to those with sleep disorders as 'patients' because I don't see them as being sick or afflicted in any way. In fact, some of them come to me having spent several nights in sleep laboratories wired up to recording equipment that hasn't thrown up any obvious neurological basis for their nocturnal problems. Some of them have also been prescribed medication that hasn't helped at all and, in some cases, has exacerbated the problem and given rise to daytime grogginess, which leaves them feeling drained and depressed.

The link between creativity and enhanced dream states and REM sleep is an important one. Many people medicate their creativity because they feel their behaviour at night is pathological in some way, without realising that there might actually be a gift buried in this so-called abnormality. My preferred approach, as always, is to help people to understand why they are experiencing these 'symptoms' and then to give them simple tools that very effectively help them to tap into their creativity and at the same time stop the strange nocturnal behaviours. No medication needed.

In fact many important scientific insights were arrived at during the dream phase of sleep. For example, Einstein dreamt that he was riding on a beam of light and from this deduced the Theory of Relativity. The physical chemist Kekulé dreamt of a snake curling back in on itself and swallowing its tail and thus discovered the ring-like structure of hydrocarbons such as benzene. A famous author, while travelling on an American Airlines plane, had a dream of being captured by a crazy woman and held hostage in a cottage in the wilderness. She tied him to a bed and broke his feet to stop him escaping. The author woke up, wrote the dream on a napkin so that he wouldn't forget it, as he knew he had a great storyline; it was Stephen King's *Misery*.

> **Experiencing bizarre dreams and sleep behaviours suggest you may be holding back or repressing your creativity. There's an important message here: What is it that you need to express?**

So the highly active REM sleep state is vital for so many reasons: we dream and create, make sense of our emotional world, consolidate memories, learn and store information, tidy our mental filing cabinets and working memory. It is important that we get enough of this type of sleep at night but too much can leave us feeling tired and drained, as if we haven't slept at all. We also need deep sleep. We need pure, sattvic sleep. Unfortunately we don't always get it.

Typical Sleep Problems

Years ago, when I started talking to people about how they were sleeping, I learnt pretty quickly that I wasn't alone and that many people were experiencing similar problems. This reassured me (as well as strengthened my resolve to solve my sleep problems and discover a way to help others).

Recently I worked with a group of high-ranking leaders and CEOs and I asked this same question, 'How are you sleeping?'

One of them replied in a slightly embarrassed tone, 'I keep waking up at 3.40 a.m. and I just can't get back to sleep. It's been going on for months now and it's driving me mad.'

I could see and feel his relief when I told him that he was experiencing one of the most common sleep problems. He too felt reassured to know that he wasn't alone. So if you're worrying that your sleeping problem is yours and yours alone, trust me when I say that you are most certainly not alone, and here's a list of some of the most common sleep problems:

- Difficulty getting to sleep or sleep initiation problems.
- Difficulty staying asleep or sleep maintenance issues.
- Sleeping but feeling as if you're not sleeping (mentally busy, 'tired but wired' sleep) – this is called paradoxical insomnia.
- Oversleeping or hypersomnia and still feeling exhausted.

- Restlessness and restless leg syndrome (RLS).
- Parasomnia such as sleepwalking, sleep talking, nightmares, night terrors, teeth grinding (bruxism).
- Delayed sleep phase syndrome – can't get to sleep until late (midnight or 2 a.m.). Technology often plays a big part here.
- Circadian rhythm sleep disorder – typically due to shift working.

Broken Circadian Timer

Sometimes when people describe their sleep problems I immediately get the sense that their circadian timer is 'broken'. Typically these are people who've never had problems sleeping in the past but something has happened – events or a change in lifestyle – that has affected the working of their timer. You may remember, this is the part of the brain in the pineal gland that controls the sleep cycle (*see page 45*). This is typically the case with:

- shift workers
- mothers (and fathers) experiencing repeated nights of disrupted sleep due to wakeful babies and children. (I'm convinced that lack of sleep is a contributing factor in postnatal depression in women.)
- addiction patients who have been using alcohol and drugs to induce sleep and the circadian timer has 'switched off'
- habitual night owls

Over the years I've done a lot of work with shift workers (as well as once being married to one) and have worked with police officers, ambulance workers, long-distance lorry drivers, train drivers and pilots. The problems I see in my clinic are many and varied, including emotional instability (for example, anger, depression, irritability), excessive alcohol consumption, high intake of caffeine and stimulants, and health problems associated with loss of physical fitness and vitality.

I also see cognitive impairment, and in one particular case the occupational health department of an airline referred one of their respected pilots to me. He was known for his sharp mind and intelligence but had repeatedly failed the flight simulation tests the previous year. When I saw him it was clear that the effect of working shifts had taken its toll on his body, mind and ability to sleep.

The effects of shift working, and particularly night-shift working, on health are well documented and studies have found that working against the body clock is detrimental to health – particularly past the age of 35. Shift work has been linked to higher rates of type 2 diabetes, heart attacks and cancer.[13]

More recently studies at the Sleep Research Centre in Surrey have shown that working shifts disrupts the body at the deepest molecular level. The study, published in the *Proceedings of the National Academy of Sciences*, followed 22 people as their body was shifted from a normal pattern to that of a night-shift worker. Blood tests showed that 6 per cent of our genes are linked to the circadian timer. However, in shift workers this genetic control of phasing is lost.[14] This may also explain why jetlag makes us feel bad, but you can see how repeated or long-term shift working can affect the body and mind detrimentally.

The ancient sciences have known for thousands of years that our bodily rhythms are connected to the natural rhythms of the universe. For example, the phases of the moon can affect your mood and emotions, hence the term 'lunacy'. It is now well documented with credible statistics that the crime rate increases during the full moon phase. REM sleep and dreaming also increase during the full moon phase and we may experience more wakefulness or disturbing dreams.[15] Anecdotally, I've noticed how patients at the clinic seem more unsettled during this time too.

So now Western science is starting to provide evidence for what Eastern science has known for some time and the studies on shift working have provided much of this validation. Professor Derk Jan-Dijk, a fellow researcher at Surrey University, describes every tissue in the body as having 'its own daily rhythm', but with shifts this perfectly synchronised rhythm is lost so that the various organ systems in the body end up in a state of what he aptly described as 'chrono-chaos', with the heart running to a different time to the kidneys running to a different time to the brain.[16]

Chemically Induced Sleep
(Why Sleeping Tablets Don't Work)

A few weeks ago I was working with a group of three patients. We talked about medication – between them they were on more than 15 different drugs: Citalopram, Mirtazapine, Pregabalin, Zopiclone, Ambien, Quetiapine, Omeprazole, Diazepam and more. One of the patients, Charlotte, was admitted to the hospital two weeks before when a sudden and traumatic death in her family three months earlier stopped her sleeping. She described feeling as if she 'hasn't slept a single night' since then and has been admitted to the hospital for a month. She's now on three types of medication to help her sleep and the drugs are starting to work, but she's exhausted. I sense there's a bright, sparky person in hiding. Her words: 'I can't feel who I am any more because of the drugs.' We spend the rest of the session talking about how to trigger the body's natural and innate sleep process and we run late because the group are thirsty to know more. Charlotte comes up to me afterwards to share just one word – 'relief'.

Important Note

Most of my patients and many of my clients are on sleeping tablets to resolve the type of sleeping issues described above, and my advice is **never to suddenly come off medication** but to work to restore healthy sleep while gradually reducing dependence on the drugs. This is my advice to you too, if you have been prescribed sleeping tablets. It may well be that you have become so out of balance and sleep deprived that your doctor has deemed that you need the help of medication.

Studies show that over time sleeping medications simply don't work but your brain may be tricked into thinking that they do. One analysis conducted by Consumer Reports Best Buy Drugs found that, on average, sleeping pills help people fall asleep sooner by just 8–20 minutes and increase total sleep time by only 3–34 minutes.[17] They also discovered that most sleeping pills actually cause poor, fragmented sleep but because they also induce amnesia you might not recall how poorly you've actually slept. Evidence of this poor sleep might be waking up feeling groggy and almost hung over. Most importantly, they don't address the underlying cause of your insomnia, nor do they give you the pure sleep that your body really needs and that you are going to learn how to access with the FAWA formula.

As I said right at the beginning of this book, your body is amazing and has all the intelligence to create your sleep biochemistry. In fact, Deepak Chopra in *Creating Health* describes the human body as 'the best pharmacy ever devised. It produces ... everything manufactured by the drug companies, but it makes them much, much better.'

This is my belief too, but some changes need to be made in order for this to happen. Keep reading. I promise this will come later.

Chapter 4

East Meets West

'In the modern world of medicine and healing, East and West have become separated, yet everything is connected.'

Barbara Wren

As I described earlier, when I returned from Australia I was looking for the answer to the deeper questions to resolve my sleep–energy issues so I turned to the Eastern sciences. I wanted to understand how and why the yoga, breathwork and meditation I was practising were bringing about such profound healing in my mind and body. Often I would laughingly joke that I'd swapped medication for meditation. I noticed that these practices were not only helping me to feel calm, relaxed and more able to sleep deeply, but also seemed to be bringing about healing at a deeper level – in my relationship with myself and others (particularly my family) and my ability to deal with big life traumas.

I wanted answers that would help me to help others too. What really happens during pure sleep that is so vital for our health? How can I help my clients and patients to get more of this? How can I solve their sleep problems, even the most complex ones? Can I work even more deeply to help them live with extraordinary energy?

I began to learn more about vibrational medicine, which is an approach to the diagnosis and treatment of illness based on the idea that we are all unique energy systems. In other words, you and I can be considered complex, sophisticated bundles of energy. All energy oscillates and vibrates at different frequencies so the human body is really composed of different types of vibrating energy – hence the term 'vibrational medicine'.[18]

The concept of the body as a complex, energetic system is part of a new scientific worldview that is gradually gaining acceptance in the eyes of modern medicine, as practices that work directly with this energy system – such as acupuncture, reflexology, homeopathy, herbal medicine and more – are now being recommended by many mainstream medical practitioners alongside traditional Western medical interventions.

What I learnt by exploring these ancient practices is what I have so far been referring to as 'vibrant energy' or 'life force'. In Eastern medicine the word *kundalini* is used to describe a latent dormant form of this vibrating energy and *prana* refers to the life-giving force of the breath – as in Hindu-based yogic practices. In Traditional Chinese Medicine (TCM) it is referred to as *chi* or *qi*, and is the vital energy that circulates around the body in currents.

TCM and Ayurveda

TCM is considered the oldest, most continuously practised, professional, literate medicine in the world. Written records date back to over 2,000 years, although the medicine is believed to go back even further. Some experts believe that TCM is at least 5,000 years old and is still practised today. Ayurveda has also been around for thousands of years. Many recent studies have demonstrated that practices, which are based on these ancient sciences, such as yoga, meditation, mindfulness, chi kung and tai chi, can bring about a measurable improvement in sleep.[19,20,21]

Whatever we choose to call our life force, the truth is that we live in an energy-abundant world. All around us is energy. Everything is energy. We are energy and the life force that flows through us is energy. We even relate to each other through our energy, whether we, or others, are dynamic or lacklustre.

A Holistic Approach to Sleep and Energy

Both Western and Eastern sciences offer holistic ways of looking at how we live our lives, and how who we are as human beings affects our health and wellbeing. Both types of medicine indicate that the different phases of deep sleep rebalance the mind and body by working on different organ systems and emotions (see Table 3 below). So you can see why these holistic sciences appealed because I have always sought to address sleep problems by looking at the whole person in relation to their whole life.

Deep sleep phase	Organ system	Rebalancing process
9–11 p.m.	Thyroid, adrenal glands	Rebalances metabolism and energy levels, replenishes energy depleted during the day. Reduces stress hormone levels. Emotional rebalancing: hopelessness, confusion, paranoia
11–1 a.m.	Muscle and tissue repair, immune system	Growth hormone production. Emotional rebalancing: bitterness, resentment
1–3 a.m.	Liver detoxification, heart and other organs to lesser extent	Emotional rebalancing: fear, anger, frustration, rage
3–5 a.m.	Lungs	Release of toxic waste from lungs (hence early morning coughing in smokers). Emotional rebalancing: grief, sadness

Table 3: *Deep sleep phases and their associated healing effects*

In Table 3 the five sleep periods in a typical night's sleep are shown. To remind you, each period consists of the five layers described previously (*see page 52*) – two phases of light sleep, two phases of slow wave or deep sleep and a short 10–15 minute phase of REM sleep. It is in the deep sleep layers (9–11 p.m.) that the majority of healing occurs and, according to TCM, each sleep period heals a different organ system in the body so habitually missing out on certain phases of sleep can cause different physical and emotional imbalances, and I see evidence for this in my clinic too.

Night Owls

Burnout, adrenal and thyroid issues and chronic fatigue tend to affect night owls, as they are missing out on this initial pre-midnight phase of sleep. They may also find it hard to get up in the morning and feel mentally foggy, or have difficulty concentrating during the day. To help them keep going, they often resort to stimulants and/or refined sugars.

Worryingly, I am now seeing a lot of younger people, and particularly teenagers, who are spending too much time on their electronic devices at night-time and then skipping these sleep phases. I recently conducted a survey of almost 500 children at a local secondary school and found that over 25 per cent of them were having sleep problems due to using technology in bed at night. Even younger children seem to be now spending more time in front of computers in the evenings, thus delaying their ability to slide into the first stage of the sleep cycle.

Sad and sleepless

Those suffering with depression typically wake in the early hours and miss their 3–5 a.m. sleep, which is vital for rebalancing sadness and grief.

Over-sleepers

Often combined with going to bed too late, in this scenario the person misses the first sleep phase, sleeps late into the day and typically feels tired all the time. Bowel function and digestion are sluggish, they suffer from poor appetite until later in the day and then overeat. They often feel stagnant and stuck in life, lacking in motivation and purpose.

Angry, Impatient, 'Liverish' and Active Addiction

A toxic lifestyle of too much alcohol and caffeine overloads the third phase of deep sleep (vital for liver and major organ rebalancing). Many addiction patients who are in rehabilitation and recovery begin to heal when they start getting deep cleansing sleep and their mood improves and they start to feel calmer and more settled.

Delving Deeper, Working Deeper

As I worked on healing my own sleep problems I began to see that while some sleep problems could be solved by adjusting our environment, behaviours and habits, others seemed to be lodged deeper our system and, as such, required tools that worked more subtly and in a different way.

I began to sense that in order to work effectively I needed to go deeper and right into the source of the sleep problem. I use the word 'sense' because this is exactly what was happening – I was sensing exactly where the sleep problem was coming from in the person's body and then finding a technique to work exactly on that area.

For example, a client would come in and I would immediately feel their scattered energy, which I describe as 'ungroundedness', and they would describe their inability to settle at night, racing thoughts and restlessness. Someone else would tell me that they were avoiding sleep, almost feeling afraid to go to bed, and I would sense a loneliness, sadness or fear. I could tell that others were sensitive human beings and needed help in understanding how to stop their sensitivity from affecting their sleep.

TCM and Ayurveda

It was my forays into TCM and Ayurveda that offered me two fascinating theories that I knew could take my work to the next levels – the theory of the *Shen* and *chakras*. I began developing and using sleep techniques based on these ancient theories and getting results, and I became even more convinced. Many of these practices may be new to you but trust that while they may not be mainstream they have been shown to work. You will learn about these practices later and, more importantly, I will show you how to use them later in the book, but first a brief overview of the theories that have proved so important in my work.

Introduction to the Shen

In TCM disturbances in your sleep might be called 'Shen disturbances'. The Shen is best translated as the spirit of the person in a non-religious sense and many forms of TCM treatment – acupuncture, chi kung, herbal medicines, Chinese massage – are focused on calming the Shen. This might sound complicated or even esoteric, so allow me to simplify; when you look at someone you might sense that their Shen is not in

73

their body. In other words their energy and attention are somewhat scattered or somewhere else. You can sense it immediately and you might say, 'You're not listening to me!' And they're not – their Shen is displaced and it might be still in the office or at school or lodged in their inbox (what a nightmare!). I see this all the time in corporate auditoriums where there is a collective Shen displacement and I have to work to bring my audience back into the room and into their bodies. When the Shen is displaced we can't sleep or our sleep is restless and 'out there'. To sleep deeply we need to be in our body.

> Some of the most effective tools you'll find in Parts III and IV work on calming this scattered energy or calming the Shen.

Everything that happens during the day is carried into your sleep, especially if you're sensitive. The feel and the energy of the day can seep right into you so that when you finally get into bed it is still there with you in the trillion of cells of your body – an accumulation of stored memories and feelings from the day. How you felt when you woke up first thing in the morning – agitated and anxious or grateful and looking forward to the day ahead. How you felt, as you got ready for work – rushing or relaxed? As you drove to work and navigated the traffic … As you opened your inbox … As you made that phone call … As you thought about your elderly mother … As you worried about your errant teenager … As you sat in yet another frustrating meeting … And so the day goes on. And so life goes on.

Remember, sleep problems are not created when you put your head on the pillow at night.

All of these experiences are held in the body as energetic vibrations and can displace the Shen. When you start to pay attention to your body, you really start to feel them. The problem is that we often don't want to consciously feel, so we distract ourselves with noise or playing on a device or checking a phone. But that vibration is still within your tissues and cells, within your energy field. Practices such as chi kung and tai chi work by helping to realign and rebalance the Shen by moving chi energy through the body. Like yoga these practices include healing postures, special movements, breathing techniques and meditations that are designed to replenish healthy chi energy and discharge impure or toxic chi – just as one would exhale carbon dioxide, the end product of normal metabolism.

Introduction to the Chakra Energy System

In Indian science or Ayurveda the energy centres of the body are called chakras. There are seven main chakras (*see Figure 2 on page 77*) that comprise our complex energy system and without them the physical body could not exist. Each chakra is like an energy wheel that spins at a particular frequency, with the lowest frequency in the root chakra at the base of the spine and the highest at the crown chakra at the top of the head. These energy centres enable us to derive our balance and determine our 'state of consciousness' or how we perceive the world.

Consciousness

Consciousness is both the most obvious and the most difficult thing to understand and define. Antonio Damasio, author of *The Feeling of What Happens* and Professor of Neuroscience at the University of Southern California, defines consciousness as 'the key to a life examined, for better and worse' and what allows us to 'develop a concern for other selves and improve the art of life'.

I recently conducted a poll of over 100 people on social media asking just this question, 'What is consciousness?' and the responses ranged from 'being aware' and 'being awake' to more complex spiritual interpretations. One of my favourite definitions came from a child who said consciousness is 'what I know'. I have extended this to 'what I know that I know'.

So consciousness is what our mind is aware of and what we know that we know. But there is so much else going on in the mind, without us even being aware of it, and this is the unconscious – what you know but don't know that you know! It is a commonly quoted statistic that we only consciously use 3 to 5 per cent of our brainpower. The rest is of the show is run by the unconsciousness.

The journey of becoming a more conscious human being therefore is about becoming more aware of how you are thinking, feeling and behaving so you can make better choices.

The chakra system itself comprises what can be thought of as your subtle energy system, and each chakra functions like a computer hard drive storing the memories of specific emotional and spiritual experiences.

Unfortunately, this can create physical imbalances and illnesses if we choose distraction over dealing with the stressful events in our lives. The energy of these events can become lodged or stuck and create energy blockages or disrupted energy flow. Information from the work of respected medical intuitives such as Caroline Myss describes how ancient doctrines, yogic chakra theory and TCM have given rise to a therapeutic model in which each chakra can be correlated with specific illnesses.[22] This is a complex concept and one that many Western scientists and clinicians still struggle to understand. However, the fact remains that many therapies and treatments, such as acupuncture, homeopathy and reflexology – which are based on this notion of energy flow and the chakra system – can and do bring about significant healing even in the most severe and life-threatening illnesses.

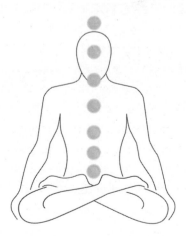

Figure 2: *The chakras or energy centres of the body*

The philosophy and science behind the chakra system is vast but for the purposes of the FAWA formula I just want to highlight the significance of each chakra in relation to sleep disturbances. Each has a colour and is associated with issues of living. As I started to work more with energy, I began to perceive how disturbances or blockages at each chakra level could give rise to the problems I was working with in my consulting room:

Root and Lower Chakra Disturbance

The first two chakras are red and orange respectively. These are where we energetically experience fight-or-flight or living in SURVIVAL mode (*see page 44*) and the energy clean-up phase of the FAWA formula works very specifically on these lower chakra disturbances. Imbalance at this level results in ungroundedness, restlessness, wired, mind racing, restless legs syndrome. The issue of safety and sleep is particularly strong; we don't feel safe enough to sleep and will often have sleep-avoidant behaviours or even addictions due to living in the base chakra, or SURVIVAL mode.

Solar Plexus Chakra Disturbance

This chakra is fiery yellow and is associated with personal power. The sensitive person taking in other people's stuff, fearful and anxious, fear of going to bed, unable to detach from problems with others. Disturbances at this level leave us literally disempowered and worrying about everyone and everything at night. The Shen is very displaced and we might even experience gastric problems such as acid reflux, which results in disturbed sleep or repeated waking.

Heart Chakra Disturbance

The heart chakra is green and is the centre through which we experience love. Imbalances here are associated with going to bed with sadness and grief, feeling lonely and unsupported, unable to let go and trust life, unable to accept help.

Throat Chakra Disturbance

The fifth chakra is sky blue and located in the throat area and is associated with personal expression. Imbalances here are related to us being unable to speak up and express truthfully, creatively blocked, vivid disturbing dreams, teeth grinding, nightmares, sleepwalking and talking.

Crown and Higher Chakra Disturbance

These chakras are indigo blue and violet. Typically here we are ungrounded and unable to switch off at night and experience exhausting and vivid and creative dreams. I also see a lot of sleep disturbances at this level with highly sensitive and empathetic people who are unable to switch off at night.

Healing Practices

Practices such as yoga incorporating breathwork, postures and movement, meditation and sound through the chanting of mantras are oriented towards rebalancing and clearing blockages in the chakras and encouraging the healthy flow of energies through them.

For some this description of the Shen, chakras and energy blockages may resonate and explain how you have been thinking and feeling. For others, the idea of a sleep problem being related to subtle energy imbalances may seem somewhat alien – particularly if you've never come across Eastern theories before. However, my aim as always is to be practical, and when you get to the Deeper Tools in Part III (*see page 139*) I'll introduce you to some weird and wonderful techniques that work powerfully on overcoming sleep disturbances. I just ask that you keep an open mind and see what happens.

So here you have the theoretical basis for the work I am going to do with you. I have shared with you Western and Eastern perspectives, which don't fight with each other, but rather offer complementary insights into the magical process of sleep. These insights have enabled me to deepen my understanding and thereby work more deeply on others and myself and I am so excited to be able to do the same for you.

So now it's time for your consultation with me – your Personal Reality Check.

Chapter 5

Your Personal Reality Check – Who Are You?

'When we peel back the layers over and over again, we are able to find the wisdom and truth of our being, the essence that we are here to share.'

Rebecca Campbell

There are so many factors that can influence how you sleep but sometimes we get so caught up in what's going on in our lives that we just can't see what's going on. Now it's time to put yourself at the centre of your life and think about what might have been affecting your sleep, your energy levels and your life.

To help you do this I am going to ask you to reflect on some questions. Your answers are designed not just to give you information but also clarity, so that you can understand your own story. I hope that by reflecting on your answers, and then linking them with the sleep theory that I shared in the previous two chapters, many connections will begin to fall into place.

- How have you been sleeping recently?
- Do you find it difficult to get to sleep?
- Do you find it hard to stay asleep – waking in the early hours (usually 2–4 a.m.) and then find it hard to get back to sleep?

- Do you worry about going to bed (for example, feeling fearful about not being able to sleep)?
- Do you feel as if you are half awake/half asleep all night? Thinking all night?
- Do you feel restless at night, as if you just can't stop moving your legs?
- Is your sleep refreshing or do you wake up feeling exhausted even if you've slept for 7–9 hours?
- Do you wake up feeling as if you haven't slept at all, even if you've slept several hours?
- Have you been experiencing nightmares or night terrors?
- Do you grind your teeth at night? Or wake up with tightness in your jaws?
- Do you worry about how much sleep you are or aren't getting?
- Do you feel if you could just get more sleep you would be able to cope better with life?
- Does the moon (and particularly the full moon) affect your sleep?

This last question is very interesting and can help you understand what type of sleeper you are.

What Type of Sleeper Are You?

In my first book, *Tired But Wired*, I described two extreme types of sleepers:

- Sensitive Sleeper
- Martini Sleeper

The chances are if you are reading this book you are currently a Sensitive Sleeper. I began using this label many years ago when I realised that many people, like me, are very sensitive in terms of their relationship with sleep. If you're a Sensitive Sleeper you wake at the slightest noise; you have to sleep on a certain side of the bed; you might travel on aeroplanes with your own pillow or blanket. You might also be very sensitive to the conversations you have before you go to bed and find it hard to let go of the day and sleep if you're feeling stressed.

I've noticed that Sensitive Sleepers tend to have certain personality traits, which you might find it helpful to reflect on.

- Perfectionists, and find it hard to relinquish control.
- Hard on themselves.
- Might grind their teeth at night or clench their jaw.
- Tightness in their neck and shoulders, as they often take on too much.
- Very sensitive to other people's energy and moods and a tendency to over-empathise.

On the positive side, Sensitive Sleepers are often great healers or therapists, highly creative and imaginative human beings.

The Martini Sleeper – and I know I'm showing my age in using their famous slogan – can sleep 'any time, any place, anywhere'. Martinis don't know why I have a job! But I remind you, being able to sleep easily doesn't necessarily mean that you're getting pure sleep, and many Martini Sleepers wake up feeling exhausted.

If you're a Sensitive Sleeper, have you always been this way or has it been more recently that your sleep has become this way? Some people are sensitive from birth but that doesn't mean you have to stay that way forever. I used to be a Sensitive Sleeper but now I am more Martini-like in my sleeping. Over the last few months I have slept in a busy Central London hotel, a tipi in the mountains of Portugal, and last summer my daughter and I slept on a slope in a field in the Peak District. We both slept deeply, despite spending most of the night rolling into each other, and woke feeling refreshed albeit a little stiff.

You might also be someone who once slept well but is now having problems sleeping due to life events and stresses. In other words: a Martini Sleeper who has become a Sensitive Sleeper. Take heart: it is definitely possible to get you back to your former good sleeping ways, if you were once that way.

Thinking About Your Lifestyle

I described earlier how every thought and emotion creates energetic vibrations in the body (*see page 75*), so this next set of questions is vital in understanding the root cause of your sleeping issue.

- What is going on in your life?
- What has been happening lately in your life?
- Are you happy at work?
- Do you work long hours? And work on the way to and from work?
- Are you happy in your close relationships?
- Have you been through something upsetting or traumatic recently?
- Have you experienced any major life events, such as moving house, sitting exams or getting married?

- Are you experiencing any other symptoms or medical problems?
- How are you looking after yourself?
- Are you exercising regularly?
- Are you eating healthily?
- How much water do you drink throughout the day?
- How many caffeinated drinks do you have a day?
- What time do you have your last caffeinated drink?
- Do you eat breakfast?
- Do you snack during the day? If so, what sorts of snacks? Are they healthy or highly processed?
- Do you crave sugar or junk foods at certain times and/or particularly in the evening?
- What is your relationship with technology?
- Do you spend a lot of time on your phone and/or email?
- Do you sleep with your devices beside you at night?
- Do you look at your phone during the night?
- Do you take breaks from technology during the day?
- What is your body telling you?
- Do you suffer from tightness in your neck and shoulders? Or do you have any other back problems?
- Do you delay going to the lavatory because you get so caught up in what's on the screen?
- Do you forget to eat?
- Do you find yourself holding your breath or sighing a lot throughout the day?
- Are you experiencing a lot of headaches?

Understanding Your Energy

You've learnt about SURVIVAL and SAFETY energy (*see page 44*) but I'd like you to think about how your energy levels feel right now.

- How has your energy felt recently? If you had to give yourself a score out of 10, where 10 is feeling energised and 1 is feeling exhausted, what score would you give yourself?
- Are your energy levels low in the morning? Does it take a long time to get going?
- Do you press the snooze button several times before you're able to get out of bed?
- Do your energy levels drop mid-afternoon? If so, do you still feel able to concentrate and perform well at any given task? Or do you feel exhausted?
- What are your energy levels like early evening when it's time to finally relax?
- Do your energy levels lift in the evenings just before going to bed? Do you then find it hard to get to sleep?
- Do you need tea, coffee or other caffeinated drinks to get you through the day? If so, how many?
- Do you feel you have the energy to do the things that you really care about?
- Are you tired at the weekends?
- Do you feel if you had more energy you would feel/live differently?
- What do you believe about sleep?
- Do you know that your beliefs about sleep can affect how you sleep?

In my experience, many people have unhelpful beliefs about their sleep and these beliefs actually stop them sleeping or affect the quality of their sleep. I'd like you to reflect honestly on the following questions, trusting that even as you reflect on your answers you are starting to work on getting better sleep.

Unhelpful Belief #1: I Can Catch Up

Do you go to bed late and then sleep later in the morning in an attempt to make up for lost sleep? Or perhaps, sleep more at weekends or when you go on holiday?

The timing of your sleep is key because while you can catch up lost sleep to some extent you can't fully recover it (*see page 64*). For this reason, it is important to get into a good regular sleep routine so that you're not missing out on all of the vital aspects of healing that sleep brings.

Unhelpful Belief #2: I Shouldn't Wake Up During the Night

Do you worry about waking up during the night, perhaps feeling that you should just put your head on the pillow and not wake up until the morning?

Well, even if you do sleep like that, the chances are that you woke several times during the night without realising it.

Sleep studies show that the average human being wakes approximately 10 times during the night. The theory is that this sleep–wake cycle evolved for our survival and safety: we come into a semiconscious state to check that all is well and we are safe and then slide back into sleep.[23] It is completely normal to wake up and maybe even need to go to the lavatory. What is not normal is to wake up, check the time/emails/

social media notifications/share prices and then to stay wide awake and fretting.

Unhelpful Belief #3: I Need to Know the Time

Pay attention to this one because this is one of the biggest disruptors of sleep. Do you wake up (which is normal) and then check the time?

If so, you may then calculate how many hours of sleep you have left, how many hours you might not sleep, how you might feel the next day and the likely implications if you've got a big event the next day (*see also unhelpful belief #4*). If you check the time and then slide effortlessly back to sleep then it's not a problem, but if checking the time obsessively is keeping you awake, why do it?

Unhelpful Belief #4: If I Sleep Badly It Will Affect My Performance Tomorrow

Do you ever have problems sleeping on Sunday night or the night before an important event?

It is often the case that the more we try to sleep the less able we are to do so. I sometimes work with elite athletes and once worked with a Premiership footballer, who (understandably) felt worried the night before playing a big game for England. I advised him to forget about sleeping the night before a game and instead focus on resting in bed. He was more able to do the latter, and before long he would fall asleep.

I also asked him to recall the number of times he'd slept badly before a big game and still performed well the next day. He was able to remember several occasions when this had happened and this also helped to take the pressure off his sleep. You too might recall that you've had nights when you haven't slept well and still passed exams and interviews or given a great presentation.

Unhelpful Belief #5: I Need 7–8 Hours of Sleep to Function

Do you fixate on how much sleep you are/aren't getting, to the extent where you might even be measuring your sleep (*see also unhelpful belief #6*)?

While I am a great believer in getting enough sleep, we often place great significance on the Holy Grail of 7–8 hours of sleep. Our sleep requirements are affected by so many factors and the key is to pay attention to how you feel when you wake up. If you wake up feeling refreshed after just 5 hours of sleep then you're probably getting enough sleep for you.

On a recent camping trip with my daughter we slept on average 5–6 hours a night but we always woke feeling refreshed and invigorated and have noticed how being in nature is in itself restful.

Unhelpful Belief #6: It Is Useful to Measure My Sleep

This is related to everything I've already highlighted and is especially relevant if you are a Sensitive Sleeper. Measuring your sleep is just going to make you more anxious about how much sleep you are or aren't getting and most measurement devices (the market is flooded with 'smart' devices at the moment) aren't actually that accurate, let alone helpful.

To sleep well you need to let go, trust and relax and not measure, control and calculate.

Unhelpful Belief #7: Sleep Is What Happens When My Eyes Are Closed

Come on – be honest! How many times have you sat in boring meetings with your eyes open, but glazed over and completely oblivious to what's being said? Or read a book before bed and then reread exactly the same pages the next night? Or stared at a TV show, with nothing going in at all, in a strangely relaxed and hypnotic state, or wanted to close your eyes just for a split second while driving (which of course you must never do)?

In all of these examples, you could be in an early sleep state – and yes, it is possible to sleep with your eyes open. I described earlier how the 'hypnagogic trance' is a vital relaxation state that enables you to consolidate information, learn and refresh the working memory thus enabling you to stay sharp and focused (*see page 56*). It's worth knowing this quirky sleep fact because you may not realise that you are actually falling asleep in front of the TV, which could be affecting your ability to fall asleep when you get into bed later, and a 'smart', sleep-measuring device isn't capable of measuring this strange type of sleep.

Unhelpful Belief #8: I Shouldn't Nap During the Day or I Can't Nap

Do you tend to avoid napping during the day, feeling that it might stop you sleeping at night-time?

Some of the world's best thinkers were prolific nappers. I positively recommend napping to everyone and especially those who have great difficulty falling asleep. It's particularly useful if you've developed a fear of going to bed because you've been having problems getting to sleep or if your sleep has been especially 'tired but wired'.

I find that a napping can almost help to reprogram your body to rest, relax and let go. It also helps to *de*-excite the nervous system so that you're not so exhausted and wired at night. But napping must be done with caution, and when you get to the Deeper Tools in Part III you'll find out exactly how and when to nap for maximum benefit.

> Everyone can learn how to nap and if you think you can't nap it's probably because you don't fully understand what a nap is (and what it isn't).

Unhelpful Belief #9: Insomnia Runs in My Family or My Sleep Problem Can't Be Fixed

You're not alone if you believe that you are somehow carrying a 'bad' gene. No such gene exists and it's more likely the belief that you are somehow carrying a 'bad' insomnia gene that is creating a big part of the problem. When you start becoming more aware of your sleep, you'll start to see how any sleep issues are probably due to bad habits that have been passed down through generations rather than faulty genetics.

People also come to see me wearing their sleep problem like a badge of honour. This might sound odd but they hold on to this strong belief that nothing will help them. I recently spoke on the phone to a doctor who'd been struggling for years to sleep. I could hardly get a word in and she spent the whole time telling me why nothing would work. She'd tried many things and I could really see why she'd be frustrated and cynical but it was also apparent to me that she'd tried each intervention with a belief that it wasn't going to work. She had a strong, intelligent mind but it wasn't working for her in this regard.

Stay open to the possibility that you can change your relationship with sleep – even if you don't entirely believe it at this stage.

Unhelpful Belief #10: I Need to Take Sleeping Tablets

This is a big one. As I described in the previous chapter (*see page 65*), please don't think I'm telling you to come off any medication that you're currently on. In fact, if you've been advised to take medication it may be for very sound reasons and coming off it could cause problems. However, I would ask you to keep an open mind as you turn the pages. You may learn about things, small things, which you're not doing and have never done but that could be the turning point for you. Very soon you are going to find out exactly what these things are – and much more.

I've described the most common limiting beliefs that I come across regularly in my work, but there are many more. I call them 'limiting' because they stop us from getting the sleep that we not only need and deserve but that we are capable of having. You may not believe this right now – because you might be sleeping badly and relying heavily on sleep medication – but it is possible.

The FAWA formula is here to help you to wake up your ability – the ability to access deep and pure sleep.

And I am going to invite you to do this by starting to work with the 5 Non-negotiables. Are you ready?

Part II
Waking Up: The Energy Clean-up

'The journey of a thousand miles begins
with a single step.'

Lao Tzu

Chapter 6

Cleaning up Your Energy
with the 5 Non-negotiables

'Healing can only occur with a surplus of resources.'
Chris Sritharan

When I first started doing this work, I used to be quite tough on my clients and felt frustrated when they came back to see me and nothing had changed – they still weren't sleeping, even though I'd shown them what they needed to do. I soon learnt (when they stayed stuck) that this approach was misguided and now know:

We cannot heal unless we are in a resourceful state and have the energy to do the work that will bring about healing.

This first programme will help you to create this resourceful state by cleaning up and recalibrating your energy, and this will shift you from running in SURVIVAL energy to sustainable energy or SAFETY mode. In a sense it is the most important programme, as it will prepare you to use the other programmes to refine and deepen your sleep so that you discover your vibrant energy.

I remind you that I call this tool 'Non-negotiable' because I really want to convey the importance of not neglecting these seemingly small but significant techniques.

Don't be tempted to fast-forward to the Pure Sleep and Energy for Life programmes because these techniques won't work as effectively unless you've cleaned up your energy first.

You will begin to notice positive changes to your sleep and energy levels very soon after you start using these five tools, including:

- Shifting the nervous system from SURVIVAL to SAFETY.
- Reducing stress hormone levels.
- Reducing reliance on stimulants such as caffeine.
- Reducing dopamine levels.
- Priming the circadian timer.

How to Use the 5 Non-negotiables (5NNs)

With my other programmes I recommend a lighter touch, but this requires a tougher combination of discipline and determination. Notice when your saboteur is telling you 'I could never do this' or 'I've never been able to do this.' This resistance is probably an indication that this is exactly what you do need to do.

You might find it easiest to start by reading through the whole chapter, then get working on the 5NNs straight away and keep going for at least 7–10 days.

Here they are:

- **NN#1:** Eat breakfast every day within 30–45 minutes of rising.
- **NN#2:** Drink 2 litres (3½ pints) of water (preferably alkalized) every day.
- **NN#3:** Reduce your caffeine intake or abolish completely.
- **NN#4:** Start an electronic sundown 1 hour before getting into bed.
- **NN#5:** Aim to get at least four pre-midnight sleeps per week.

The first three NNs are particularly important because they very quickly fire up the circadian timer, but let's look at each one in detail.

Non-negotiable #1: Eat Breakfast Every Day within 30–45 Minutes of Rising

When I was at university, I have no idea how I managed to pass exams and do well because at that time I was struggling with my sleep and energy levels. Breakfast was coffee and a cigarette. The thought of it makes me feel sick now, but back then my energy was so different. My life was so different too and I was running in SURVIVAL.

I'm sharing this with you because I see so many people who struggle with eating breakfast and I do understand it. However, this is the strategy that could make the biggest difference to your sleep and energy levels. This is my most important Non-negotiable and is related to what you know now about the SAFETY/SURVIVAL energy systems (*see page 44*). Eating breakfast stops you relying on your survival system (SNS) and switches on the safety system (PNS) in which your circadian timer can be activated and switched on.

In this way you'll start to make more of the sleep hormone melatonin and, in so doing, sleep better. Eating breakfast stabilises your blood sugar levels; the famine state is broken (hence the term 'break-fast') and you won't need to rely so heavily on the stress hormones to keep you going. Do this for just three days and see what a difference it makes to your sleep.

To summarise, people who eat breakfast (and people who don't experience the opposite):

- Tend to have less difficulty falling asleep and staying asleep.
- Wake up with more energy in the morning.
- Are less inclined to press the snooze button.
- Are less inclined to wake up feeling anxious and more likely to wake in a good mood.
- Have less reliance on caffeine first thing in the morning and throughout the day.
- Tend to have a more efficient metabolism and are therefore less prone to weight gain.
- Tend to have a reduced post-lunch afternoon energy dip.
- Tend to wake up feeling hungry and wanting breakfast.

This last point is important. You might feel as though you can't eat in the morning because you're not hungry in the mornings. When you start eating breakfast, your metabolism will kick in and you'll wake up hungry.

How are you feeling about this? Are you feeling those stir-rings of resistance and defence of old behaviours or are you looking forward to trying this out? I'm really hoping it's the latter because I know the difference it will make for you. Here are some of the common questions I'm asked about eating breakfast:

I thought you were going to help me to relax and sleep. Why are you telling me about breakfast?
Your pattern of eating affects your blood sugar levels. Not 'breaking fast' lowers your blood sugar levels, which informs your brain that you are living in famine. The brain reads this signal as being a crisis and switches on the SNS and stress hormone production. Conversely, eating breakfast informs your brain that you are living in a world where there is enough food – which it reads as safety – and switches on the PNS and sleep/energy systems. It's as simple as that.

I haven't eaten breakfast for years. Why should I start now?
If you always do what you've always done then you're likely to get the same results again and again. Ask yourself, how are you sleeping? How are you feeling? What are your energy levels like? Is what you are currently doing working for you? If not, isn't it time to try something different?

I'm a busy working mum with three children to get sorted before I leave the house. How can I find time for breakfast?
I hear this a lot from busy people. My answer is that if your life is hectic and busy then you especially need to eat to fuel the demands of your day. I'm not talking about sitting down to a luxurious three-course meal. If life is busy then shovel your porridge in while you're on the go. It's not ideal but eat while emptying the dishwasher, feeding the cat, checking emails, making packed lunches, putting the washing on,

blow-drying your hair. In case you haven't realised it, I'm describing how my mornings sometimes look! It's important not to get caught up in the potent tide of adrenaline energy, which will probably get you through your morning but will leave you feeling flat and exhausted later in the day and then unable to sleep at night.

Is eating breakfast when I get to work good enough?
Not really. For many people the journey into work is stressful – driving in traffic or rushing to get to a train station on time, competing to get a seat, pushing through ticket barriers, rushing past people on escalators. It is not a peaceful experience and your faithful adrenal glands may already be running in overdrive and chucking out adrenaline to get you through this ordeal. Eating before your journey will stabilise your blood sugar, give you energy and prepare you biochemically to produce melatonin later in the evening. You may even find that your experience of your journey is somehow less stressful.

Should I eat breakfast within 30–45 minutes of getting out of bed or actually waking up and lying in bed?
When you wake up, does your mind immediately begin racing, planning ahead and rushing forwards into your day thinking of all that you need to do? The speediness of your mental chatter is an indicator that your body is already starting to run in overdrive and on adrenaline, which means that you need to get up and eat as soon as you can. If you're lying there relaxing and snoozing peacefully, then you can probably wait until you're fully awake and out of bed.

Isn't my latte enough, if I have lots of milk in it?

No. You need to eat before having any caffeine so that you stabilise your blood sugar and stop any activation of the SNS (which caffeine does). Even if your drink is very milky, you'll still experience the full effect of the caffeine on your nervous system. Check the caffeine buzzometer (*see page 110*) to learn more about how caffeine affects the body and how much caffeine there might be in your favourite beverages.

If I start eating breakfast, will I put on weight?

On the contrary, eating breakfast will actually increase your metabolism by up to 10 per cent, and this effect can last for hours after eating. This is called the 'thermogenic effect' and it's a bit like putting fuel into a fire and getting a bigger fire. So, in effect, eating breakfast is a very healthy weight-control strategy.

What if I exercise first thing in the morning?

If you exercise within 30 minutes or so of rising, then you might prefer to eat breakfast after your session. But it's important to eat within 20 minutes of completing your exercise session in order to replace the muscle glycogen used. This will help maintain your energy throughout the day, as well as keeping your metabolism high following the exertion.

What about if I do yoga or meditation first thing? I'm not supposed to eat before my practice.

This is the other exception. When I'm on a yoga retreat or even on holiday, I might eat a little later as my body and mind are in a completely different state of balance. In fact, in Ayurveda it is recommended that you fast for a few hours in the morning and wait for your digestive fires, called *agni*, to ignite and build. I love doing this on retreat and really notice the health benefits on many levels. However, when I'm back in the Western world and running at full pace, my SNS is more active and there are more demands on my energy and time. There are different strategies that I need to adopt in order to maintain balance in this world, and eating breakfast soon after rising is one of them.

Are 'breakfast biscuits' a good choice?

Unfortunately, these are usually marketed as 'healthy' nutritional options but often come loaded with saturated fats and refined sugars, which will cause a big spike in your blood sugar levels, leaving you feeling hungry and depleted before long.

Is there something small I can eat just to get started on this?

This is my 'eight almonds and two dates' principle. This small portion of food will fit in the palm of your hand, contains roughly 150–200 calories, and contains the perfect combination of protein, fat and carbohydrate and is enough to help break the 'can't eat breakfast' cycle. You will need to eat something more substantial 90–120 minutes later but it's enough to get your metabolism going, stabilise your blood sugar, stop you reaching for the coffee (and a cigarette) and help you produce that vital melatonin later in the day.

The Breakfast Everyone Can Eat

When my late father was diagnosed as diabetic and struggled to eat breakfast in the mornings, preferring instead a couple of virtually 'solid' cups of coffee, I'd say to him, 'Dad, just try eight almonds and two dates.' Being an engineer, he liked knowing the exact number he was required to eat and it also stopped him eating the whole packet of nuts and dates, which would have been very harmful to his blood sugar.

If you want to learn more about breakfast and other options – after all, living on almonds and dates will start to become very uninspiring after a while – take a look at my website (http://www.drnerina.com) for some breakfast ideas, my very special granola and energy bar recipes. For now, the tiny portion size of the almonds and dates will help to break the cycle of being unable to eat in the morning.

As you continue using NN, you'll find that your metabolism increases over time and you start feeling hungrier in the mornings. The amount of time it takes for this effect varies from one person to the next but if you keep going for 21 days (*see page 36*) you should be able to introduce more substantial and delicious breakfasts before long. For me now, it's often the thought of breakfast that gets me out of bed in the morning whether I have to catch an early flight or it's a day in the office after the school run.

Are you ready to adopt the first NN? What are you going to eat for breakfast tomorrow morning?

Non-negotiable #2: Drink at Least 2L of Water per Day (Preferably Alkalised)

The body is made up of over 70 per cent water and, remarkably, this accurately reflects what we see in planet Earth's geography with the ratio of land to ocean. We are a reflection of nature and a part of nature, and this is something that I return to time and again when helping people to sleep. This return to nature is the key to our return to our innate ability to sleep. You will learn more about this later, when we begin to explore some of the powerful sleep tools, but for now let's examine our natural relationship with water.

Many of us are living life too fast and, as a result, are in a state of dehydration. Living life too fast speeds up all of the cellular systems, and in particular the kidneys. Drinking too much caffeine exacerbates this speed and dehydration effect, as does spending too much time in centrally heated, air-conditioned environments, and eating food that has been artificially flavoured and processed, refined and stored, resulting in loss of natural water content. In her book *Cellular Awakening*, Barbara Wren also describes in detail how mobile and digital phones, computers, Wi-Fi and even electric blankets all create potentially harmful fields of electromagnetic interference within our cell membranes, leading to dehydration. She also describes how this 'dehydration alert' can send us into stress and fear mode – the opposite of being able to sleep.

Did you know that your brain tissue holds the highest water content of any tissue in your body – being 80 per cent water? So, when we are dehydrated, our brain is the first organ to register this deficit and the regulatory systems in the brain that control sleep are thrown out of kilter.

TCM offers a fascinating perspective on the importance of being hydrated because it is understood that fear and stress are held within the element of water. This element controls and sustains the kidneys, brain and central nervous system, so if you are feeling stressed and fearful, these vital organ systems are often the first to be affected and this in turn affects your sleep. So you can see that if you're in a job that you hate or choosing to remain in a relationship that's making you unhappy this will affect your body cellular systems and, ultimately, your sleep. The solution? Drink more water.

Like the 'eating breakfast' solution, many people balk at this suggestion. Common complaints range from 'I hate the taste of water' to 'I'll be rushing to the bathroom too often' or even 'Have you heard of that person who died from drinking too much water while running a marathon?'

Trust me, dying of over-hydration – a condition called hypernatremia – is extremely rare. So rare, in fact, that when it happens it tends to make the news. The 'rushing to the bathroom' concern is an understandable one but, again, I can reassure you that if you start gradually you will eventually build up more muscle tone in your bladder and will be able to hold more fluid without feeling any urinary urgency. The walls of the bladder are made of muscles and any muscle, if exercised regularly (in this case, by stretching), will become more toned and elastic. Floppy bladder muscles do not make for good retention.

If you don't currently drink much water then start gradually by drinking ½–1 litre (¾–1¼ pints) of water per day and build up slowly until you're drinking at least 2 litres (3½ pints) per day.

To ring the changes, go for dilute fruit squashes or juices, herbal non-caffeinated teas, or add flavour to your water with mint leaves, slices of fresh ginger, lime or cucumber.

As regards not liking the taste of water, I really can't argue with this other than to say that if you had the choice between getting used to the 'discomfort' of drinking more water or sleeping beautifully and living with bountiful energy then perhaps it's a bit of a no-brainer?

Alkaline Water

In recent years there's been a lot said about the value of alkaline diets and alkalising methods, and I have to say it's not all quackery. Now if you're already drinking water and want to take it to the next level then you might want to experiment by adding just a squeeze of lemon juice and a tiny pinch of natural sea salt. The citric acid in lemons is, of course, acidic, but inside the body – once the lemon juice has been fully metabolised and its minerals dissociated in the bloodstream – its effect is alkalising.

As a physiologist, I learnt many years ago that the body functions optimally at an alkaline pH of around 7.35. Every one of your 75 trillion cells needs to be bathed in a fluid held at around this pH in order to function at its best. This is because our cells run on four main electrolytes – sodium, potassium, calcium and magnesium. These electrolytes create charge in and around the cells and the existence of this charge moves water in and around the body. The movement of this water enables the cells to transmit messages freely around the body, thus enabling all our physiological processes including nerve transmission, hormone secretion and cellular responses to environmental stimuli such as light and dark. All of which are vital to our ability to switch on the circadian timer – and sleep.

Don't forget that this book is also about energy. You will notice that your energy levels will also increase once you start drinking more water. The energy currency of the cell is called adenosine triphosphate or ATP. The four electrolytes are key to moving energy in and out of the cells and, again, this process is hydration- and pH-dependent.

It would be easy to discount such a simple strategy as drinking more water. But trust me, it can make a huge differ-

CLEANING UP YOUR ENERGY

ence. My patients who begin to adopt this strategy no longer experience restlessness at night and report that the 'noisy scratchiness', as a client aptly described it, of their sleep disappears.

Non-negotiable #3: Cut Out or Reduce Caffeine

How much caffeine are you drinking? Do you really need that cup of tea or coffee first thing in the morning to get you going? Or in the afternoon to pick you up? And how have you been feeling lately?

Medical recommendations would stipulate that you can get away with about 400 milligrams of caffeine per day; however, it's important to understand what that means in terms of cups and types of drinks.

When I wrote *Tired But Wired* I included my caffeine buzzometer, which many people found very helpful. Then my research indicated that most coffee shops were serving people drinks that contained at least 10 times the amount that they might have in their home brews. In doing the research for this book I found it more difficult to come up with a definitive caffeine guide, as the levels vary so much from one coffee-shop brand to another. But I have found that caffeine levels have increased since compiling my first buzzometer and it was one day while sitting in a café that I realised why, when I listened to a customer order a grande cappuccino with three extra shots. He looked tired and grey, and I wondered how he might be feeling later in evening when it was time to sleep. So, if you want to know much how much caffeine you might be consuming, these are the typical levels I've found.

Cup of instant coffee	80–100mg
Cup of homemade filter coffee	150–200mg
Cup of commercial coffee (e.g. Costa or Starbucks)	350mg
Cup of tea	40–80mg
Green tea	20–30mg
Cup of cocoa	10–20mg
Can of cola	30–50mg
Can of energy drink	80mg

Table 4: *Caffeine levels*

Many people ask for 'extra shots' in their favourite brand but, even if you don't, it seems that the coffee shops have responded to the demand by upping the level of caffeine in our drinks. I now make a point of asking 'How many shots are in my drink?' and then asking for less or for some of the shots to be decaffeinated.

But what's the big deal about caffeine? The link between caffeine intake and health risks is well documented but here are a few things to consider in relation to sleep:

- The half-life (time taken to drop to half the concentration in your blood) of caffeine is 5 hours, which means if you have a caffeinated drink at 5 p.m. you will still have half the amount in your blood supply at 10 p.m. This might not make you feel energised but it may be enough to stop you getting to sleep or going into those vital deep sleep levels.
- Caffeine blocks the action of melatonin.

- Caffeine stops the breakdown of adrenaline in the liver, and higher adrenaline levels stop you sleeping.
- Caffeine increases the number of times you wake during the night and the amount of REM sleep.
- Caffeine steers your nervous system down the SURVIVAL route and switches off the PNS.

I have clients who drink several cups of coffee or tea a day and still sleep, but they tend to be very tired and look pale or grey, so clearly they aren't getting deep, nourishing sleep.

So How Does This Non-negotiable Apply to You?
If you're drinking more than four or five caffeinated drinks a day then you're definitely in a fatigue cycle. Halve your caffeine intake, start eating breakfast if you're not already, increase your water intake and start snacking healthily every 2 hours or so to maintain your blood sugar levels. You may experience uncomfortable withdrawal symptoms if you withdraw caffeine without maintaining your blood sugar in some other way, so choose from the following snacks to stop you reaching for that cup of coffee:

- 8 almonds and 2 dates (or equivalent – some cashew nuts and raisins, or Brazil nuts and dried figs)
- 2 rice cakes and 2 tablespoons of cottage cheese
- 1 small pot of full-fat Greek yoghurt topped with chopped nuts
- 1 piece of wholemeal toast with nut butter
- A few slices of Parma ham and crackers
- A few oatcakes with hummus or half an avocado

And,

- Avoid any caffeine after 3 p.m.
- Don't drink a caffeinated drink before you eat breakfast – this will just send you down the SURVIVAL energy route, which will affect your sleep later.
- If you can, and you're really committed to getting amazing sleep and energy, cut out caffeine completely.

This principle might be difficult for you but you will really feel the benefits. Keep reading the book, as you'll continue to learn more about how to truly nourish your energy levels in a sustainable way and, by doing so, won't need the quick-fix cure of caffeine. The intention is to start listening to your body. To listen to its whispers before they become cries and to work out what it is trying to tell you. Why are you reaching for a cup of coffee or tea? Do you need to eat something? Or take a break and move? Drink some water? Breathe more deeply?

Ask yourself, 'What is it that you really need?'

Non-negotiable #4: Electronic Sundown 1 Hour before Bed

As I described in Chapter 3 (*see page 46*), our energy tends to run in 60–90-minute cycles and the cycle before going to bed is absolutely key to how you are going to sleep when you get into bed at night. Unfortunately this is the time when you may find that your brain has suddenly woken up and you find yourself unable to switch off – particularly if you've been bombarding your brain with blue light and technology. The effect of the dopamine will keep you alert and switched and it suppresses the action of melatonin.

This Non-negotiable is about switching off and withdrawing from technology in that hour before bedtime. How do you do that when for so many it has become such a habit? I recommend that you start in small ways thinking very consciously about how you are connecting to technology. For example, while you're watching TV, do just that – watch one screen only. The norm these days is to dual and triple screen and multitasking has become a way of life for most of us. It's so hard to do just one thing. So you might sit there watching something on TV that doesn't require much mental effort while at the same time doing your shopping and keeping an eye on your social media feeds and emails. All of this is possible these days, isn't it? But what is it doing to your brain and how does it affect your sleep later?

When you surf the net or check your emails the chemical dopamine is produced, which makes you alert and switched on.[24] It's actually called the 'reward' or 'wake-up' chemical. So you sit there trying to concentrate on the sitcom plot and your phone buzzes or pings and you mentally respond with an 'Ooh, I wonder what that is?' Even though it might not be anything of significance, you find yourself continuing to hold your device, gliding your fingers over the screen and looking for something you might have missed or just mindlessly following links on the Internet without realising that you don't even remember what you were looking for in the first place.

Here's the neurophysiology of what has just happened. The blue light has suppressed the production of melatonin from the pineal and at the same time activated the SCN (the part of brain that tells us it's time to wake up). Cells in the hypo-thalamus secrete dopamine, which wakes you up, telling you it's time for action. You get up to go to bed and realise you're wide awake so you decide to check your emails and social media feeds. What makes it worse is if, at some point in the evening, tiredness led you to doze just a little bit while watching TV. Even if you were dozing with your eyes open, you will have used up some of your sleep debt. The combination of these biochemical reactions deactivates the circadian timer – so you lie there in bed and simply can't get to sleep.

Do you also use this dopamine effect to get you going in the morning? These days most people reach for their phones as soon as they wake up, and research conducted by Dr Alvaro Pascual-Leone,[25] a professor of neurology at Harvard Medical School, showed that the level of brain activity that is stimulated when someone picks up their phone in the mornings is similar to what you'd see if you'd had a cup of coffee.

This isn't just about falling asleep and sleeping but also about waking up with amazing energy, the right type of energy.

Non-negotiable #5: Four Pre-midnight Sleeps per Week

My final Non-negotiable is about getting to bed before midnight. Ever heard the old-fashioned saying that an hour before midnight is worth two after? There's a lot of sense in this as your best quality of sleep is obtained when your circadian rhythm is at its lowest point (usually between 10 p.m. and 5 a.m.). Therefore, even if you obtain a good amount of sleep (7–9 hours), going to bed late is likely to lead to a large amount of your sleep being highly inefficient. And you read in Chapter 2 about pure sleep that the phase before midnight, according to TCM, is the phase when levels of stress hormones start to drop off and we get a substantial hit of deep sleep and our shortest phase of REM sleep. This phase is deeply nourishing and, if vanity is a good motivator for you, it's incredibly anti-ageing. As Barbara Wren says in her book *Cellular Awakening*, 'To remain balanced, open and healthy, we each need to be able to dance with the rhythms of nature.' She also describes the period before midnight as being 'a time of high energy to cleanse at a deeper level'. So it seems this is an important time for cleansing and detoxifying the body on many levels.

If you struggle with this one because you're a bit of a night owl, start to get into the habit of reducing stimulation and becoming quiet and restful during this time. You don't have to be in bed and fast asleep by 10 p.m., but resting, avoiding technology and blue light (*see Non-negotiable #4*), withdrawing your senses, letting go of the day and preparing your mind, body and spirit to sleep. You may have got used to staying up late, but in my experience a lot of people become this way inclined because of the habits they've got into rather than having an innate night owl rhythm that runs their circadian timer. You may also find that once you've started using the other Non-negotiable strategies you are more able to find it easier to get to bed earlier because your physiology actually begins to change.

This is an important part of the FAWA formula because, apart from the deeply restorative sleep you're getting here, I have noticed that when people begin to follow this strategy it begins to create a different attitude and mind-set towards their sleep. A different kind of mindfulness and awareness of what is happening in their body that previously went unnoticed. Many of us actually start to feel sleepy around 9–10 p.m. but we override this signal by adopting the unhelpful behaviours I've mentioned so many times already or actually dozing off and using up our valuable sleep debt.

Head up to bed earlier, start to power down and get ready to rest. Over time you will begin to really notice that you're feeling relaxed, drowsy and actually looking forward to getting into bed. This is a strategy that I recommend even for those clients and patients with a long-standing history of insomnia and they often start to see a difference within 7–10 days.

Many people seem to have lost the art of 'turning in' early and I'm often asked, 'What do I do if I go to bed then?' They are so used to being on their devices or being engrossed in endless episodes of their favourite box sets and they don't know what to do with themselves when they remove these crutches. Here are a few suggestions:

- Read a relaxing book – nothing too over-stimulating or exciting.
- Write a gratitude journal just simply listing all the things that have happened in your day that you are grateful for (*see page 157*).
- Meditation in the earlier part of the evening. Avoid meditating just before going bed as this can actually energise you, making it difficult to actually sleep afterwards (*see page 199*).
- Do a few minutes of pre-sleep yoga or progressive muscle relaxation, such as my 'pre-sleep 5-minute yoga routine' (*see page 161*).

- Sketch or doodle.

Whatever you choose to do, make sure that it is relaxing, helps you to feel safe and secure and helps you to come back into your body and out of the mental chatter.

Over to You

So there you have it – the 5 Non-negotiables. Do them for the next 7–10 days or, even better, 21 days. Be determined. Make a plan and stick to it. Tell your family and friends what you are doing. Stick a note on your fridge door or bathroom mirror reminding you what you're aiming for. Post it on social media and get people to support you. Most importantly, make it imperative – remember WHY you're doing it – pure, deep sleep and an abundance of vibrant energy.

Living not surviving.

Part III
Fast Asleep: The Pure Sleep Programme

'Sleep is the best meditation.'

The Dalai Lama

Chapter 7

Introducing the Tools in the Pure Sleep Programme

'Sleep is that golden chain that ties health and our bodies together.'

Thomas Dekker

By now you may be starting to see how sleep issues aren't simply due to whatever happens when you place your head on the pillow but are affected by the myriad choices you make during the day. The Pure Sleep Programme is designed with this in mind and the tools I'm going to share with you next will help you to assess these choices and whether they are helping or hindering your sleep.

The tools have been organised specifically to work from outside in. In other words, the first set of techniques, the **Essentials,** works on your external behaviours and influences – such as the choices you make during the day, before going to bed and in relation to your sleep environment. The focus of the next set of techniques, the **Deeper Tools I** and **II,** is more internal and will help you to become aware of the inner choices that you are making – thought patterns, mind-sets and inner dialogues – that are affecting your sleep without you even knowing.

Using these tools, you will start to become more conscious of the unconscious patterns you've built up that are disrupting your sleep and draining your energy. In this section I will give you what I consider to be the **Ultimate Deeper Tool**. This tool is simple but so effective and I promise that, if you use it in the way I recommend, it can change your life. That's a grand claim to make but, trust me, I have witnessed this countless times in my work so I feel totally confident about making this assertion.

The **Deeper Tools** are divided into two sections (I and II) and the difference between them lies simply in the depth at which the techniques work. By using the techniques in Deeper Tools II, you will be working with the more subtle disturbances in your energy that can give rise to sleep problems. So if you can, imagine these tools as drilling down deeper and deeper to the true source of your sleep and energy problems.

Chapter 8

The Essentials – Preparing to Let Go

'By letting go it all gets done.'

Lao Tzu

In East Meets West (*see Chapter 4*) I offered some Eastern perspectives in which I described how everything that happens in the day – the vibrations of the day – seep into our body and can affect our sleep. Using the following simple Essential tools will help start to smooth out the energy and agitation from the day and so lay the foundations for sleep. Many of the following techniques are what might be called 'sleep hygiene' (and you may have tried some of them). They are important because they prepare us to let go of the day – to forget, for example, that worrying email or conversation or the angst you experienced when running late for a meeting – and send an important message to your primitive, childlike brain, the state we go into before we go to sleep (*see Chapter 3*), that you are safe.

Empty the Mental Filing Cabinets

Going to bed with the worries of the day in your mind won't help you to sleep. You will either feel as if you've a mad monkey in your brain – the classic 'tired but wired' sleep – or you may find that, even if you do fall asleep, you wake in the early hours with the same worries plaguing you.

To let go of the day before bed, simply get a pen and paper, and write a list of what needs to be done tomorrow. Get it all out on paper. Ideally write this list before leaving work, or a couple of hours in advance of bedtime, so that you can really leave any work worries behind you. Just by doing this you are preparing to enter the next compartment of your life – home.

> If you use public transport, you might choose to use some of your journey time to write your to-do list.

Case Study

One of my clients was a Family Liaison Officer in the police services. His work involved offering support to the families of victims and, understandably, it could be extremely stressful at times. He'd moved house so that his long commute was now a mere 20-minute drive. However, he found that he would arrive home still carrying the stress of the day so he took to stopping in a quiet spot on the way home, simply sitting there for 10 minutes or so and allowing the worries of the day to diffuse out of him before he saw his family.

Even 10 minutes of transition time like this can help you to let go of the day. It brings you back into your heart, reminding you what's important and what isn't. Too many of us go home carrying the worries of the work day with us. Look about and you'll see it on the faces all around you – they've physically left but mentally they're still at work. No wonder so many people find it difficult to engage with their families when they get home. No wonder they can't sleep.

As I've described in Chapter 4, the Shen becomes displaced if we spend too much time in our heads and not enough in our hearts (*see page 73*). In order to fall sleep and enjoy restorative sleep, we need to bring the displaced Shen back home. In other words, we need to come out of our heads and back into our hearts.

If your mental filing cabinets are crammed with worries about family members, present challenges or fears about the future, then again spend a little time writing these down before going to bed. You might even start a special journal specifically for this purpose. Write down every single thing that you're worried about. Don't hold back. In the early, quiet hours, these worries can be transformed into nightmares and night terrors by the creative unconscious. In the middle of the night even minor worries become magnified and scarier than they need to be.

> Ideally write your lists in a different room to the one you sleep in and well before retiring to bed. Your bedroom, after all, should be your sanctuary.

Bringing your worries into your conscious mind – giving them the space and time they need – is a way of acknowledging that you know they are there. You're allowing them to take their rightful place in your conscious mind, not in your deepest dreams.

Creating a Sleep Sanctuary – Sights, Sounds and Smells

Look around your bedroom and feel how the space feels. If you're not in your room, close your eyes, take a deep breath and imagine it. Ask the following questions:

- How does it feel?
- How does it smell?
- What does it look like?
- What noises can you hear around you when you lie down to sleep?
- Does it make you feel peaceful, at ease?
- Does it make you feel safe?

This is about using your unique senses to work out what is right for you. Creating a sleep sanctuary is particularly important if you're a Sensitive Sleeper (*see page 83*) for whom sights, sounds and smells are prime considerations.

I'm inviting you to feel your sleep space. Is it cluttered and untidy? Are the colours restful and peaceful or clashing and overstimulating? Do you have visible signs of work in your bedroom – piles of books and papers, a laptop or other electronic devices? Do you have a TV in your bedroom? Are piles of laundry or children's toys in sight?

Your bedroom should be a place of rest and relaxation so the first step is to declutter and tidy it up. Ensure that work, the laundry basket or children's toys are firmly out of sight. If the last thing you see before shutting your eyes reminds you of your daily life then obviously it will be harder to leave the day behind and enter deep sleep. The same goes for TVs, laptops and mobile devices, so remove them from your bedroom.

> Watching TV, surfing the net or catching up with your social media feeds in bed isn't conducive to getting peaceful, deep sleep so I would strongly advise against it.

What about the temperature in your room? There is an optimum temperature for good sleep – ideally around 19° centigrade (66° Fahrenheit) – but remember, this is about how you feel and what you need. There is a similar argument for the level of darkness in the room – what makes you feel safe and able to rest and let go? Some sleep experts might recommend complete darkness and blackout blinds or curtains. Feel into this for yourself – you will always come up with the answer that is right for you, if you take the time to ask the question.

And what about the smell of your room? You may not even realise it but the smell of your bedding and bedroom can help or hinder sleep. Experiment with aromatherapy oils and find the ones that are calming and soothing to your senses. Again, this is highly individual. For example the soporific and relaxing scent of lavender is widely reported, but do you like the smell of lavender? If not, don't use this oil. It's as simple as that.

Personally I love a combination of lavender and eucalyptus oils and always have a small bottle of each on my bedside table. My attachment to eucalyptus oil comes from the fact that my mother used a lot of eucalyptus-containing chest rub ointment when I was a child and so I associate it with her – and feeling safe and comforted. I now take a bottle everywhere I go – when I'm staying in hotels, on long-haul flights and even when I go camping.

What scents do you associate with feeling at home and safe? Experiment with different oils or diffusers until you find one that evokes a sense of relaxation and peace.

Feng Shui

The Eastern art of *feng shui* (pronounced 'fung shway') has been practised for thousands of years in China and in the last 20 or so years has gained popularity in the West too. Feng shui takes the approach that your surroundings affect not just your level of material comfort but also your physical and mental health, your relationships, and your worldly success.

Feng Shui examines how the placement of things and objects within it affects the energy flow in your living environment, and how these objects interact with and influence your chi, your personal energy flow (*see page 75*). Your chi flow affects how you think and act, which in turn affects how well you perform and succeed in your personal and professional life.

In organising our homes we often intuitively follow feng shui principles, and generally if your home feels peaceful and comfortable then you've probably got a lot of it right. If it doesn't then you might want to find out more about this ancient art as its common-sense principles offer a useful resource for creating a sanctuary in your bedroom.

White Noise

If you're a Sensitive Sleeper, live in a noisy environment or even if the sound of your own thoughts keeps you awake, then you may benefit from having some form of white noise in your bedroom. White noise is a bland, continuous noise that can block external sounds or changes in your environment, such as traffic or a dog barking, which might otherwise wake you up. The shallower your sleep, the more susceptible you will be to night awakenings, and a source of white noise in your bedroom can help stop the intrusions.

The simplest white noise machine is a fan but you can also buy machines, which are specifically designed for this purpose, and play the sounds of the rainforests or the sea, for example. There are numerous white noise apps available for downloading onto your phone or laptop, but devices in the bedroom is contrary to one of my most important Non-negotiables (*see page 112*), so go for the next best alternative: a white-noise track set on repeat on a CD or music player (not your phone).

If you are thinking, 'I could never do this. Having sound in my room while I'm trying to sleep would drive me nuts,' think again and just try it. Have a short 20-minute nap/rest during the afternoon (more on napping later) with a fan on in the bedroom and notice how it affects you after a few tries. You may find that the white noise becomes less of an intrusion and more a trigger to let go and relax.

You may recall that I mentioned right at the beginning of the book that after decades of using one I no longer need my fan in the bedroom. Keep experimenting with the programmes, and you too may eventually find that you are sleeping so deeply that you are no longer so easily disturbed and, if you are, are able to fall asleep again with ease.

Case Study

One of my patients was at the clinic for recovery from alcohol addiction and used alcohol at night to help him pass out so that his neighbour's nocturnal movements were less likely to disturb his sleep. I'm not saying this was the root cause of his drinking by any stretch of the imagination but it certainly wasn't helping. Adding white noise to his bedroom helped him tune out the external noise and became part of his overcoming alcohol addiction.

Sharing Your Sleep Space

If you are a Sensitive Sleeper then sharing your bed with someone else might not be a straightforward consideration, as it can bring up all kinds of issues around feeling safe – in your level of trust, support and faith in both the relationship and yourself. Ultimately this is about doing The Real Work, which you will learn about in Part IV, but for now there are a few practical considerations that will go a long way to helping you share your space.

- Get the biggest bed you can afford and that fits in your bedroom, and make sure that the design is such that the effects of your partner's movements are minimal (single sprung mattresses tend to be the best for this).
- Consider adding some white noise to your bedroom (*see page 129*).
- There is nothing wrong with occasionally sleeping in separate caves when you really need to get some sleep, for example if you've got a big event the next day.
- If you or your partner snores then seek help from your medical practitioner to find its underlying cause.

I'm not a relationship counsellor but I often find such issues in my consulting room. After all, the root causes of sleep issues are nearly always life issues, and the key here is conscious communication and negotiation. Don't ignore the problem and hope that it will go away – talk about it. Become aware of and talk about the differences in your relationship with sleep, especially if you're a Sensitive Sleeper and your other half is a Martini. Lovingly negotiate when you will sleep together and when you can't. Know that you aren't alone with this and that this issue is remarkably common.

If, after using some of the tools in this book, you still feel sharing a cave is a problem in your relationship then there might be a case for both of you seeking professional help as the fundamental work may lie in establishing trust and safety in the relationship.

Case Study

Recently a client came to see me in tears and on the verge of giving up on her relationship because of her partner's snoring at night. She's a Sensitive Sleeper and he's a Martini, and his nocturnal snuffles and grunts were literally driving her insane. Meanwhile, her partner was struggling to understand why it was all such a big deal.

After one session she was able to go back to her partner and explain the differences in their relationship with sleep. They invested in a bigger bed and a fan. Her partner also came to see me for a session and we looked at addressing the possible root causes of his snoring, which included being overweight, dehydrated and unfit. Addressing these few issues didn't solve the whole problem but they went a long way to fixing it.

Stop Measuring

Not measuring how much sleep you get sounds like such a small thing, but is it? Many of us are so used to being in control during our waking hours that we forget that in order to sleep we need to be in a state of trust and letting go. It might seem trite, but checking the time during the night and worrying about how many hours sleep you have left is linked to something more profound – our need to keep up and manage life, when in reality there is so much in life that we really aren't in control of. I remind you of one of the beliefs I shared with you earlier (*see page 53*):

It is normal to wake during the night and we may have evolved with this pattern of waking for our very survival.

What is not normal is waking and measuring and calculating, which brings you into full, wide-awake mode, fretting consciousness and worrying, 'Is that really the time? How many hours before I need to get up? And what if I don't get this X number of hours of sleep? How will I feel tomorrow? And how will I cope with everything I've got to do?' – a small but unhelpful choice that triggers a cascade of fear. The opposite of what is needed for deep, healing sleep.

At the risk of repeating myself, no one – not even a Martini sleeper – needs to measure their sleep, whether it's by mental calculation in the middle of the night or with so-called smart measuring devices.

Case Study

A well-known Olympic athlete had huge problems sleeping before an event. The rest of the time she slept beautifully. Her sleep problems were due to a red line that her coach had suggested she draw on the wall opposite her bed – this was how high she needed to jump in order to win the gold medal in the high jump. She did go on and win gold – proving that the odd night of bad sleep really doesn't affect performance – but I wonder how much better she might have felt the night before, if this extreme form of measurement hadn't been imposed?

There are highly effective alternatives to checking the time and worrying. Keep reading – as you delve deeper into the Pure Sleep Programme, I am going to show you exactly how to use some simple techniques to help you fall asleep if you wake during the night or struggle to fall asleep.

Case Study

At a party recently a man came up to me and thanked me for helping him to sleep. He had a long-standing history of sleep problems and had tried many things but it was the 'clock' tool in *Tired But Wired* in particular that had helped resolve his sleeping issue. He'd simply stopped checking the time during the night and this small thing had made such a big difference. He still wakes up but less frequently and he's able to get back to sleep almost immediately. This successful businessman was used to being in control, and he certainly had the material success to prove it, but it was clear that a large part of his success was about being in control and perfectionism, and it wasn't working for him at night.

Once Upon a Time ...

This is where my work differs from some other sleep therapists who often say absolutely no reading in bed. Personally I can't imagine life without my bedtime book, and if you have a similar relationship with reading then you'll feel the same.

Remember, your relationship with sleep (and life) is unique to you.

So, yes, if reading relaxes you and helps you let go of the day; yes, if it helps you go to sleep thinking the world is a good place. No, if it's that must-get-to-the-end-of-the-book whodunit; no, if you're reading on an electronic reader – the blue light suppresses melatonin production (*see page 53*); no, if you're reading the news on your phone or a newspaper.

Consciously and mindfully choose the book that you read before you go to bed, particularly if you're going through a lot of stress. You need to be kind to yourself.

> The choice of bedtime story is relevant for children too – they especially need to go to bed feeling safe, so help them choose stories or poetry that have a calming effect and help them put aside any worries about the day. In times of particular anxiety, for example in the lead-up to exams, encourage them to use the list-writing exercise described earlier (*see page 124*).

Stories have a rhythm. Words have a rhythm and resonance that affects our senses and our personal vibration. This rhythm can soothe you to sleep or wake you right up, which is why you might want to keep that exciting thriller for when you're on holiday. The feelings a book evokes can leave you tense and unsettled or they can lull you to safety and sleep. The vibration of the words can take you to far-flung places in your imagination but also take you into your own deeper stories, bringing insight and realisations but also reactivating old wounds and sadness, which can then wreak chaos in your dreams.

Ultimately, to sleep deeply, you need to be with yourself and in the 75 trillion cells of your body, not in your mind.

You need to feel safe to do this, and choosing the perfect bedtime story can bring you home to safety. So, with this in mind, and particularly if you're a sensitive human being, you might want to think very consciously about your bedtime reading and how it makes you feel and sleep.

Wash the Day Off

I'm sure you've been told umpteen times that a bath can help you to relax and sleep, but why? Sure, soaking in the tub can relax the muscles and the mind but, as always, I want to encourage you to think about those energies and vibrations – the Shen (*see page 73*) – from the day that you're still carrying in your cells.

Just as you let go as you write your to-do list, so you continue the cleansing and letting-go process as you wash the day off.

Soaking in a hot bath is wonderful but there are also times when what's called for is a complete showering off of the day. I find this particularly helpful when I've been working very intensely at my clinic, and I have heard the same from those working in the emergency services – they need to shower the day off and especially before engaging with their family.

We are highly sensitive to other people's energies through-out the day, so showering before bed, even if you've already had a shower that day, is an easy way to encourage calmness and stillness within. As you start to listen more deeply to your body, you will get better at hearing what it needs.

Deeper Cleanse

For an even deeper washing off of the day, you might want to try a powerful cleansing bicarbonate bath.

1. Add 350 grams (12 ounces/2 cups) of bicarbonate of soda (also known as baking soda) or substitute with 175 grams (6 ounces/1 cup) of pure sea salt (not synthetic table salt) to your bathwater.
2. Immerse your entire body, including your head and hair, in the water for at least 20 minutes.
3. Relax deeply and focus on your breath for a few moments, before going back through your day in your mind's eye and imagining every worry of the day being drawn out of your body and into the water.
4. Rinse off with clean water afterwards.

To maximize the benefits of the bicarbonate bath,

- Don't use soap or shampoo in your bath. If you feel particularly grimy, take a shower first.
- Don't drink any alcohol before or after your bath.
- Do ensure that you are well hydrated before taking your bath and aim to drink a large glass of water while you're in it.

> You might also like to add a few drops of your preferred aromatherapy oil to the water, light some candles and play soothing music.

Be prepared to feel very tired after such a deep cleanse. You may need to go to bed shortly afterwards. Bicarbonate baths are very detoxifying, and ideally don't have more than one in a week.

The Essential tools of the Pure Sleep Programme will make a big difference to how you're sleeping, and prepare you for the powerful Deeper Tools I and II, which will take your sleep to the next dimension.

Chapter 9

The Deeper Tools I and II – Sattvic Sleep

'One conscious breath – in and out – is a meditation.'

Eckhart Tolle

Remember the Fast Asleep, Wide Awake formula is not just about getting you sleeping but about getting the pure sattvic sleep that brings about the *deepest* restoration of your energy (*see page* 4). This in turn paves the way for you to do The Real Work. So, are you ready to go deeper?

The Ultimate Deeper Tool

First let me introduce you to perhaps one of the simplest but most effective techniques that I've been teaching for all the years I've been doing this work. It's something that we all do naturally every day – breathe. In the coming chapters you'll note I will often ask you to focus on and notice your breath because it can profoundly affect your energy levels and the way you sleep. So the Ultimate Deeper Tool will help you become more aware of how you breathe so that you can become consciously better at it. Hopefully, eventually this will become an unconscious competence and you won't need to think about it so much.

Notice Three Exhalations

This first breathing technique described below paves the way for all of following techniques in this section – the equivalent of opening up the box of Deeper Tools and getting ready to use them.

1. Wherever you are right now, and without changing your posture, simply pay attention to your breathing and notice three exhalations. Don't try to change your breathing pattern or do anything fancy to it. Just allow your body to follow its own intelligence and breathe. (Note: This might feel tricky for those of you who practise yoga or Pilates because you might be inclined to judge your breath and then change it [it needs to be deeper or more in my belly, or it needs to do X, Y or Z], but the aim of this exercise is to stay neutral and just notice your breath.)
2. Each time you breathe out, silently and softly say to yourself, 'OOOOUUUT' for the whole duration of the out-breath.
3. Notice that each out-breath is different and not necessarily rhythmic or uniform.

Use this tool for a minimum of five times a day for the next 21 days.

> If you're tired and need a quick lift in your energy, use the 'notice three exhalations' tool with your eyes wide open, as closing your eyes will just make you more tired. If, on the other hand, you're feeling stressed and overwhelmed, do it with your eyes closed and notice the difference when you open your eyes.

What I especially love about this technique is that you can do it right here and now. No props needed – no yoga mat or mountaintop. You don't even have to close your eyes. Do it first thing in the morning, as soon as you wake up and even while your eyes are closed. Do it last thing at night as you drift off to sleep. Find a few times to do this during the day – queues, traffic jams, while you're washing up, stirring the pasta, before and during meetings. Just notice three exhalations.

Why Do This Exercise?

We breathe an average of 20,000–25,000 times a day and the majority of the time our breathing is unconsciously controlled. But when we get caught up with emails, have-to-dos, stress and life, we start holding our breath or taking shallow breaths. If you go through your day sighing or yawning this may indicate that you are holding your breath or breathing inefficiently. Poor breathing switches off that all-important healing vagus nerve: it activates the sympathetic nervous system, acidifies the body, increases adrenaline levels and creates tension in the upper body (*see page 24*). But most importantly:

Inefficient breathing drains your energy and stops you sleeping.

Poor or shallow breathing is associated with insufficient melatonin levels. So you can literally breathe your way into producing more melatonin. Using the exercise regularly during the day fires up the vagus nerve – called increasing vagal tone – so that when you get into bed at night this nerve is already active and ready to help take you into deep sleep.

In the Essential tools (*see page 123*) I mention not checking the time when you wake during the night (notice, I use the word 'when' because it's completely normal to wake up in the night). You can use the 'notice three exhalations' tool to get yourself to sleep or put yourself back to sleep – simple and easy.

There's another reason why noticing three exhalations is such a powerful exercise. In his bestselling book *The Seven Habits of Highly Effective People* Steven Covey talks about the space between the stimulus and the response. In other words, when we move our focus on to our breath, rather than whatever is going on in our external environment, we pause and remember that we have choice. In this space we can make more intelligent and kind decisions. We can decide whether to react angrily to our teenager, reach for another chocolate cookie or a cup of coffee, send that career-limiting email, or fire off the millions of knee-jerk, sleep-disrupting reactions that we all make when we don't stop to think.

Notice three exhalations and you create a big gap between stimulus and response, and so make better choices.

Case Study

Recently I was involved in a leadership programme and I asked the delegates to try the 'notice three exhalations' exercise. One of them, a likeable but somewhat cynical senior manager from an IT company, said in frustration, 'I just don't get this!' His logical, highly mathematical brain was expecting instant fireworks. I recommended he go away and keep using the technique for the next few weeks and let me know how he got on. Less than a fortnight later he sent an email thanking me: his wife said he was like a new man, he was less short-tempered and meetings at work seemed to be going smoother. 'By the way,' he added at the end of his email, 'I seem to be sleeping better. Is that anything to do with this breathing thing?'

Now you are ready to go deeper.

Deeper Tools I

Years ago I described this first set of tools in *Tired But Wired* but I have since developed them further, and because they are integral to the FAWA formula I've outlined them here again.

Rest and Reset Throughout the Day

In order to greet life calmly, we need to have inner stillness. At first this may require some practice. Ideally stop every 90 minutes or so for a few minutes and do something restful. Think of it as pressing the RESET button. Use it to change channels mentally, physically and spiritually. Breathe deeply – use the 'notice three exhalations' exercise (*see page 140*). Get away from screens and technology. Eat something nourishing. Walk up and down a flight of stairs. Drink a cool glass of water. Think of someone you love. Look at a picture or photograph that inspires you. Read a poem or quote that touches your heart.

> **If you've been sitting for a long time then the most restful thing might be to move. Get up and stretch.**

One of my favourite resets if I am working from home is to stroke or brush my cat. Often she'll put in an appearance just at the time when I need to stop and take a break.

Pressing the reset button regularly throughout the day changes the way you feel, as it works on several levels by:

- Emptying your working memory.
- Clearing up mental files and information so that your sleep will be purer and less noisy.
- Rebalancing the nervous system from stressed sympathetic to healing parasympathetic (*see page 45*).
- Replenishing your energy and it reminds your mind and body of that calm state that is vital for peaceful sleep.

Practise Napping

Many sleep therapists strongly advise against napping during the day as (they say) it can stop you sleeping at night. I agree that if you nap – or rather sleep – for too long and close to bedtime then this will inevitably affect your sleep. If you are a good sleeper and/or are oversleeping, then napping is not the technique for you. However, if your sleep is disturbed at night and you feel tired during the day, then powering down for 10–20 minutes at some time between 2 and 4 p.m. has a number of benefits:

- It will recharge your mental batteries so you come back to your task with increased focus.
- It helps to *de*-excite the nervous system, thus allowing for deeper, less noisy sleep.
- It helps you to rest and let go without worrying about whether you will actually sleep or not.

This last point is important if going to sleep has become associated with fear and anxiety. Resting in this way retrains the mind that sleep is no longer the enemy. This is mainly because napping really isn't sleeping – it's just resting. A nap can simply be sitting somewhere quiet – perhaps at your desk or in a quiet space – with your eyes closed and focusing on your breathing, allowing your thoughts to come and go.

When you first start napping you might fall asleep, so you might want to set an alarm. You might also feel that nothing is really happening, but you will notice the benefits – often after the first session.

If you come out of your nap feeling exhausted this is probably because *you are* exhausted and need to replenish your energy by changing your daily habits and adding in more of the following techniques and tools.

> For an even more powerful nap you might incorporate some specific rejuvenating yoga postures, such as napping with your legs slightly elevated on some pillows or up against the wall (*see page 162*). Learning yoga nidra or a form of progressive muscle relaxation while napping is also very powerful and many scientific studies have shown the impact of such napping on boosting the immune system, damping down the sympathetic nervous system and strengthening the parasympathetic nervous system, and promoting deep, restful sleep.[26]

Give Space to Your Creativity

As I described briefly in Chapter 3, parasomnia – nightmares, night terrors and vivid dreams – can be due to ill-expressed creativity (*see page 43*). The important thing here is to allow space for your creativity – and preferably not just before you go to bed because you don't want it to spill over into your sleep. Whatever form your creativity takes – writing, poetry, art, music, gardening, cooking – give it expression. If you don't this energy becomes suppressed and repressed. And it can make you ill.

For the next seven days or so try writing in a journal or sketching – even if for just 15 minutes or so – and notice the effect on your sleep.

Practise Letting Go During the Day

Sleep is about letting go mentally and physically, so practise letting go during the day, maybe on the 90-minute cycle. The tool works in the same way as pressing the 'reset' button (*see page 144*) but here I want you to really focus on letting go throughout the day and particularly after stressful meetings, traffic hold-ups or difficult discussions – anything that leaves you feeling worried or tense.

1. Say to yourself, 'I'm letting go.'
2. Check in with your body and notice whether you're holding on to any tension.
3. Check your shoulders – are they hunched?
4. Soften and relax your jaw – is it clenched?
5. Relax the space between your eyebrows, soften your gaze, relax your belly and buttocks. Scan your body and see where you are holding on.
6. Notice your breathing. Were you holding your breath? Allow yourself to breathe in whatever way feels natural. Exhale with a long sigh, AAAAAH, feeling your breath drop down into your belly.
7. Check yourself now. Has anything changed in your body since reading these last few lines?

8. You might also like to repeat the following mantra quietly to yourself, 'I relax. I let go. I allow myself to relax and let go. I am peaceful. I am safe. I let go.'

9. You may also want to write the words, 'I'm letting go,' down on several sticky notes and place them in areas where you will see them. Repeat the words to yourself, as you would an affirmation or mantra regularly throughout the day and for the next 21 days to become an expert at letting go.

Affirmations and Mantras

These are phrases or words that can help to reset our thinking. It could be something simple like 'relax' or 'breeeathe' or an entire phrase, such as 'I am letting go'. Many of those used to performing at the top of their game and with extraordinary energy, such as athletes, use mantras and affirmations to help maintain a winning and positive mind-set. And you too can use the energy of your thoughts to create healthier patterns. By mentally repeating a specific, positive word or phrase over and over again you can bring about healing benefits on a variety of physiological and psychological levels.

The use of structured affirmations and mantras in healing goes back nearly 100 years. Emile Coué, a French pharmacist, gave his patients 'conscious autosuggestions', as part of a mind/body healing experiment. The basic affirmation was as follows, 'Every day in every way, I am getting better and better.' With repetition of this simple mantra a total of 20 times every morning on waking, the patients began to feel better. His work has become the precursor to many techniques now used for stress reduction and pain relief.[27]

Letting go needs only take a few seconds – you just have to remember to do it – so practise it as many times as you can throughout the day, and especially when you are tensing up in response to something. We unconsciously accumulate so much tension during the day. We hold on in our mind and the body tenses up. We hold on in the body and the mind tenses up. We store this tension – and we take it into our sleep and then can't work out why we're so wired, and at the same time exhausted.

Case Study

After coming to see me, one of my clients, a highly perfectionistic mother of two young children, realised how much 'holding on' was draining her energy and contributing to her severe neck and shoulder tension, and restless sleep. Using a simple affirmation of 'breathe and let go' was enough to change her energy levels score from a 3 to an 8 (*see page 86*) and restore peaceful sleep after just 10 days.

The Best Mind-set for Sleep and Energy

You now know that what you believe about your sleep can in itself create sleep problems (*see page 86*) and cognitive behavioural therapy (CBT) has been found to be very helpful in challenging the limiting beliefs that can give rise to sleep problems.

'Reframing', as it is often described, the way you view your sleep or the way you talk to yourself about sleep, is as simple as changing the words you use.

To find a more positive mind-set start by examining the way you talk to yourself about your sleep and then ask, 'Are my beliefs helping me to sleep or are they creating more anxiety and worry?' Then find a different sleep mind-set by using one of the following reframes:

- Don't use the word 'sleep'; use the word 'rest'. So you might say, 'If I can't sleep tonight I will rest.'
- The night before a big event you might say, 'I can still perform well, even when I don't sleep well the night before.'
- If you are lying in bed unable to sleep tell yourself, 'I am enjoying resting.'
- If you are fearful about going to bed and whether you will sleep try saying several times throughout the day, 'I wonder if I will sleep tonight,' or 'I am looking forward to resting tonight.'
- If you want to bound out of bed in the mornings try saying, 'I am looking forward to getting out of bed tomorrow morning.'

Deeper Tools II

The following techniques work even deeper on the subtle chakra system that I described in Chapter 4 (*see page 75*) and work with your energetic body and spirit – the place where the most of the deep-seated source of sleep problems often reside. This is where techniques such as acupuncture, reflexology, homeopathy, aromatherapy, craniosacral therapy and many other forms of therapy work.

These techniques used to be described as 'alternative therapies' but now they are increasingly being recommended by medical doctors and clinicians who use traditional Western medical interventions alongside such complementary therapies to great effect.

Working with your subtle energies might sound complicated but actually these techniques are quite simple and fun. However, you may need to practise using the exercises a few times before you really start to gain the benefits from them – particularly if you've never done any form of yoga or martial arts before. Once you've got the hang of them they can be done quickly and easily.

Drawing in the Shen

To sleep deeply, we need to be in the body, not in the mind, which means the Shen needs to be in your heart and solar plexus – not scattered, as it might if you've had a stressful or over-busy day. The simplest way of describing this technique is that it draws your attention and awareness back into yourself. It is also an extension of the 'notice three exhalations' tool (*see page 140*) and can be used in so many ways:

- To help you to get to sleep.
- To help you to get back to sleep when you wake during the night.
- During power napping.
- Throughout the day to help you draw the Shen back into the body and so feel more centred and balanced.
- As an instant pick-me-up when your energy levels are low.

When using the following tool for the first time, read one step at a time and then do that step rather than trying to do the whole exercise. There are three simple steps and it can take as little as a few minutes.

1. **Awareness – noticing the scattered beam:** Close your eyes and simply notice what you become aware of when you're quiet. Do this for 1–2 minutes, then open your eyes. What did you become aware of when you closed your eyes? Were you aware of external sounds? Sensations in the body, such as tightness or your breathing or your heartbeat? Were you aware of thoughts?

2. **Drawing in – focusing the beam:** Close your eyes again and do Step 1 again but this time notice your breath. Don't try to change your breathing pattern – let it do whatever it wants to do. Just follow it using the words 'IN' and 'OUT'. Whisper these words to yourself silently. You may find that your breathing is very irregular – some long breaths and some short. Do this for 1–2 minutes and then open your eyes. Did you notice that you were more aware of your breathing and inner sensations? Even if you are still aware of external noises, your focus will have turned inwards towards your body.

3. **Lengthening and deepening – sharpening the beam:** Close your eyes and focus on your breathing again, but this time gently lengthen each exhalation – 'OOOOOUUUUUUT'. Imagine you are sending the exhalation out through your lower body, through your hips and thighs, knees, lower legs

and feet. Imagine the out-breath going all the way down into the Earth's core. Breathe back in. Don't worry about the in-breath – it will naturally follow. You may find that your breathing becomes deeper and drops right into your belly. As a result of breathing out for longer you will breathe in more fully. As you deepen your breaths, imagine drawing your energy right into your body.

Ideally practise this exercise five times a day: first thing in the morning before you get out of bed, last thing at night and then a few times during the day. During the day you might prefer to keep your eyes open and practise drawing in the Shen as you go about your normal tasks – washing the dishes, sitting in a meeting or at your computer, for example.

Once you get the hang of simply drawing your attention inwards and reclaiming your scattered energy, drawing in the Shen can be done in a minute or so and will help maintain your equilibrium and energy levels.

Grounding and Rooting

This tool is useful for those times when you're finding it hard to switch off because you're overthinking issues or can't let go of specific problems, random words or snippets of conversations. You may recognise the signs as feeling physically spaced out and not in your body.

Grounding and rooting works with the base or root chakra (*see page 78*) and will calm and ground your nervous system while bringing you right back into your body and out of the mental realm.

1. Stand with bare feet about hip-width apart. Spread your toes and feel the ground beneath your feet.
2. Close your eyes and breathe deeply into your belly, prolonging the exhalation as described in step 2 of 'drawing in the Shen' (*see page 152*).
3. Sway gently from side to side, feeling the four corners of your feet.
4. Take your awareness to your first chakra (for women, it's the space between your ovaries; for men, it's the base of the spine).
5. Imagine a green ball of light as wide as your hips sitting in this space. Drop this green ball of light down to the centre of the Earth and, as you do so, imagine it forming into a green grounding cord connecting you to the centre of the Earth.
6. Visualise little green threads of light extending from this grounding cord to your buttocks, across your back and down your legs.

Ideally use this exercise just before getting into bed or whenever you're feeling spacey, unfocused and ungrounded.

Earthing, Grounding and Rooting

This exercise builds on the previous one, 'grounding and rooting', but is perhaps most helpful when you're feeling wired and unable to switch off due to too much screen time or technology overload. You may recognise the signs as feeling hyperactive or buzzing in the nervous system.

Being in nature is one of the most effective ways of counteracting the unnatural effects of being constantly surrounded by electromagnetic radiation and feeling wired.

1. Stand on a patch of damp grass or soil with bare feet and breathe deeply in this position.
2. Use the root chakra visualisation described in steps 4-6 of 'grounding and rooting'.

The dampness helps to earth electricity from your body while grounding you at the same time. If the soil or grass isn't damp then you can water it with a watering can before doing the exercise or even stand on the grass while watering your feet. You may get odd looks from your neighbours but I promise you'll experience the benefits in your sleep and energy the following day.

Use this exercise whenever you're feeling unfocused and ungrounded and especially if you've spent hours at your desk, in an air-conditioned office and in front of a screen. This exercise can also be helpful if you're feeling unsettled after hours of travel – especially air travel.

Cutting the Cords

This is a particularly helpful exercise if you're worrying about someone, or something, close to your heart, perhaps elderly parents or children. This type of worry can leave us feeling sad, emotional and even grief stricken. The exercise works by calming the solar plexus and heart chakras (*see page 78*) before you sleep and works particularly well if used in conjunction with the gratitude exercise described next.

1. Light a candle or simply imagine a huge bonfire in front of you.
2. Sit or stand with your feet planted firmly about hip-width apart.

3. Now imagine that silvery threads connect the person you are worrying about straight into your solar plexus (the seat of your emotions and located under your ribcage) and your heart.

4. With both hands gather these cords together and pull them away from you while still holding on to them. With your right hand, make a downward chopping motion and cut the cords right out of you and throw them into the fire.

5. Play with your intuition and ask if you've really disconnected from whomever or whatever you are worrying about.

6. If there are remnants of worry remaining then repeat the exercise as many times as you need to. Each time you throw the cords into the fire, imagine them being burnt and transformed to pure healing light.

A common worry about doing this exercise is that you are disconnecting from the person in an unkind way. Trust that this is not the case and that you are lovingly disconnecting from the problem or the worry about them so that you can sleep and thus give yourself the energy and resources to help them.

> The cutting the cords technique is really helpful for children who are worrying about school or perhaps finding it difficult to let go of an argument with friends.

Use this exercise just before going to bed, at any time during the day or for getting back to sleep after waking between 2 and 4 a.m. If you wake during this time, avoid checking the time, get up to use the bathroom if you need to and then use the cutting the cords exercise before getting back into bed. Try to stay as sleepy as you can, so do it with eyes half open.

I also recommend doing this exercise if you've had a nightmare or bad dream. Don't think too much about the dream but simply cut the cords (of the dream) followed by the noticing three exhalations exercise (*see page 140*) to return to sleep. Cutting the cords in this way can stop you carrying any bad feelings from your dreams into the next day.

Gratitude

You can use this tool in combination with the cutting the cords exercise above, if you're feeling sad or if you're feeling unsafe and insecure at night – either when trying to get to sleep or getting back to sleep.

Ultimately it is about helping you to feel safe so that you can sleep, and it works with the energy of the heart chakra (*see page 79*). In drawing in the Shen (*see page 151*), you learnt how to bring energy back into your body when it has become displaced; this tool brings the Shen right back to its home in the heart.

The Shen can become displaced when you're feeling sad because it's simply too painful to feel what needs to be felt. So you might find yourself engaging in distractions – particularly those provided by technology – and then when you go to bed you feel the worst combination of being wired and also feeling a background sadness in the heart.

1. Lie in bed on your back with eyes closed.
2. Place your left hand over your heart, calming the heart chakra, and your right hand over the solar plexus just above your belly button (calming the emotions of the solar plexus).

3. Breathe deeply into your hands while silently repeating the words, 'Thank you.' Breathe into the words. Feel the words as deeply as you can. You might want to think of specific people or events from your day that you are grateful for.

4. As you say 'Thank you,' imagine that a beautiful soft rose-pink light begins to emerge from the centre of your heart.

5. See this light becoming bigger and brighter until it fills your whole body. Imagine every cell of your body being bathed by and filled with this light.

Who you are thanking depends on your beliefs. It might be God, some higher power, yourself, your family or others for making things possible. Either way, these two words – 'Thank you' – are the most powerful and healing in the dictionary, and they bring about an immediate letting go, softening and feelings of safety. This isn't about pretending that your life is perfect but simply acknowledging that there is good in your life, if you are prepared to see it, and for now you're just going to put your problems aside and remember those blessings ... and sleep.

Use this tool while lying in bed and preparing to drift off to sleep or if you wake during the night.

Speaking Your Truth

This exercise is for when you're finding it hard to show your emotions or speak your truth – which may manifest as teeth grinding or jaw clenching – or if you find yourself seething inwardly while putting a smile on your face. You may also find it useful if you often have dreams that replay stressful conversations or things you should have said. Performed regularly, this exercise can also help to alleviate snoring (*see page 132*).

This tool works on the fourth chakra, which resides in the throat area (*see page 79*) and is about expressing your truth. The yoga-based exercise is called *simhasana* or lion pose.

1. **Get into lion pose:** Kneel on the floor with knees shoulder-width apart and sit on your heels. Lift your chest up just enough so that you're not slouching and your spine is fully straightened, but don't over-arch your back. Place both your hands on top of your knees. Widen your palms and press them firmly against your knees. Splay your fingers like a lion's claws. Inhale deeply through your nose.
2. **Roar like a lion:** This next step is the focal point of simhasana. Read through the following steps and practise a few times before simultaneously doing the following steps in lion pose:
   • Lower your jaw and open your mouth as wide as possible.
   • Stretch your tongue out and curl its tip down towards your chin.
   • Open your eyes wide, looking upwards.
   • Focus your eyes in between your eyebrows or on the tip of your nose.
   • Contract the muscles at the front of your throat.
   • Activate your hands, splaying your fingers further out.
3. Now, hold this position and exhale slowly through your mouth. Feel the air pass over the back of the throat as well as the contraction of your throat and neck muscles. You should make a distinct 'haaaaa' sound as you exhale.
4. Don't forget to give your best lion roar. In fact, roar two or three times, then retract your tongue.
5. Relax your face, mouth, eyes, throat and hands.

Use this tool before bedtime or any time during the day when you feel you need to release. It's also a great exercise to use before a presentation or conversation that you're feeling nervous or unsure about.

Winding in the Telescope

If your seventh or crown chakra and your sixth or pituitary chakra – also known as the third eye (*see page 79*) – are too open, they become channels for allowing too much information in. Your sleep might feel noisy with vivid and disturbing dreams, and exhausting, as if you've been travelling all night.

This tool is for very sensitive human beings and sleepers, who have a tendency to over-empathise or be hypersensitive to other people's moods and vibrations. For example, one of my friends works as a carer in a home for the elderly and she uses this technique to help her sleep. Practised regularly, this exercise can help reduce the occurrence of very vivid and disturbing dreams.

1. Close your eyes and spend a few moments simply noticing your breath.
2. Imagine your crown and pituitary chakras like flowers (*see page 79*), fully in bloom and open at 100 per cent.
3. Now imagine them closing to about 20 per cent. Don't worry if you're not confident about being able to visualise; simply say, 'I am closing my crown chakra and third eye to 20 per cent.' And it's as simple as that.

Use this tool as you prepare to wind down to sleep or to help you cope in a noisy and overwhelming environment. You may find that you feel more self-contained and less spaced out after doing this. Your sleep should also feel deeper and less noisy.

> Children respond well to this technique if they tend to get overwhelmed at school, and it can also help to improve their ability to concentrate and focus.

Bedtime Yoga

As I described in Chapter 4, yoga has been around for thousands of years and it can have a tremendously therapeutic benefit on mind and body (*see page 69*). The following mini yoga routine works specifically to balance all of the chakras and calm the nervous system, thus enabling deep *sattvic* sleep (*see page 4*). The entire routine only takes 5 minutes or so and no props – not even a yoga mat – are needed.

I created this routine especially for a Premiership footballer who was having problems sleeping after playing in football stadiums filled with tens of thousands of noisy, clamouring fans.

Yoga is a wonderful tool before going to bed, as it is helpful in calming the nervous system when you're feeling over-stimulated from the day or when you've been working late and need to get to bed shortly after getting home.

> For maximum benefit, aim to hold each pose for at least 2–3 minutes.

1. **Child's pose** (*see Figure 3*): Kneel down on the floor and bend down to the ground with your arms above your head and palms resting on the floor. This first step brings you into the childlike pre-sleep state and helps draw your energy inwards from the day. Breathing deeply in this posture activates the vagus nerve. If you're uncomfortable in this posture or have a tight lower back, use cushions to support your forehead. Think about letting go as you rest in this posture. Repeat, 'I am letting go. I am relaxed. I am peaceful. I am safe.' Hold the pose for 2–3 minutes or for as long as is comfortable.

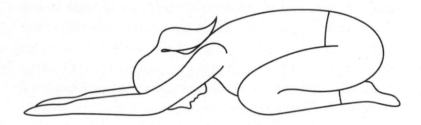

Figure 3: *Child's pose – building safety*

2. **Legs up the wall pose** (*see Figure 4*): Lie on your back with your arms resting by your sides and palms facing upwards, and then elevate your legs by resting them against a wall or other vertical surface. Elevating your legs brings about further activation of the vagus nerve, and palms facing upwards is symbolic of letting go and acceptance. Again, if there is any discomfort, use cushions, pillows and blankets to support yourself. You can also do this lying by the side of your bed with your legs over your bed or simply lying with a pillow or two under your knees. Raising your knees above the level of your heart is what deepens the experience.

Deepen the letting go process by repeating the following mantra, 'I allow myself to let go deeply and fully. I am safe.' Hold the pose for 2–3 minutes or for as long as is comfortable.

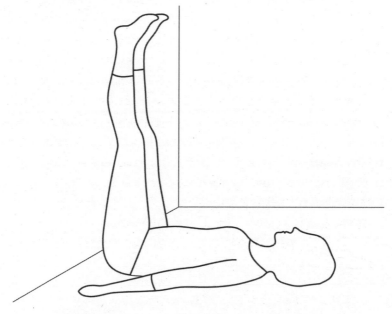

Figure 4: *Legs up the wall pose – surrender*

3. **Corpse pose or savassana** (*see Figure 5*): Lie on your back with your legs hip-width apart, feet falling to the side. Take your arms out to the side at a 60-degree angle to your body, palms facing upwards. This is the posture of deepest surrender and letting go. Repeat the mantra, 'I let go of my day. I am open to receive deep healing and peace. I am open to receive deepest rest and sleep.' Hold the pose for 2–3 minutes or for as long as is comfortable.

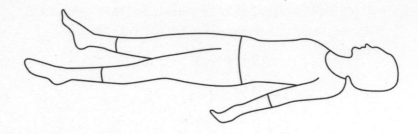

Figure 5: *Corpse pose or savassana*

So there you have it – my Pure Sleep Programme. Are you now ready to take things to the next level? What brought you to my book in the first place? What is really at the deepest core of your sleep problem? Are you ready to tap into vibrant, extraordinary energy?

If so, you're ready to do The Real Work.

Part IV
Wide Awake

'Who looks outside, dreams;
who looks inside, awakes.'

Carl Jung

Chapter 10

Doing The Real Work and Tapping into Extraordinary Energy

'Life does not happen to you, it happens for you!'

Jim Carrey

I am hoping that by now you've started using the 5 Non-negotiables together with the Pure Sleep Programme and the FAWA formula is beginning to work its magic on your sleep. Maybe your energy levels have lifted to at least 6 or 7 since you first answered the Personal Reality Check questionnaire in Chapter 5 (*see page 81*) and you're starting to enjoy the feeling that comes from shifting from survival to sustainable energy.

Maybe you're now ready to do The Real Work. If so, I am going to offer you the Energy for Life Programme, which is perhaps more of a set of life principles or life lessons. However you choose to label or use them, they can be considered an invaluable set of practical strategies that will support you in this next stage of your journey.

There are many rewards to doing The Real Work but I'm not going to lie to you, it can be hard. It means no longer running away, avoiding, medicating or distracting. It means facing headlong whatever needs to be faced – whatever was stopping you from sleeping and draining your energy in the first place.

**Maybe The Real Work
should come with a warning
on the packet because it does
take courage.**

Deep, reliable support is also absolutely essential in doing this work – I know this from both my personal and professional experience. After my breakdown, which I described earlier (*see page 31*), it became clear to me that the supports I'd created in my life up until that point hadn't been reliable. From the moment of my awakening in Australia I set out to find anchors, which would subsequently serve me whenever things fell apart. But they didn't arrive overnight in a lightning flash of insight – it took me years, decades in fact, to find ways of navigating my way through the rich, mulchy stuff of doing The Real Work.

**I deliberately use the word
'mulch' because this is the stuff,
the fertiliser from which comes
vibrant growth.**

When I had my life-changing moment in Brisbane, you might remember, there I was sitting on a sunny veranda writing my journal and sipping a latte. I looked up and something had changed. I felt different. In that moment I had this realisation that life could be different for me and that it wasn't happening to me but for me. That I was at the centre of my life and therefore responsible for what happened and no longer needed to be defined by a label (bipolar disorder). But to be honest, I wasn't quite sure at that point what I was going to do differently but I felt empowered and optimistic.

I returned to England in a wildly enthusiastic mood, expecting life to be wonderful from there on. What ensued, however, was a journey of highs and lows – although nothing like I'd experienced in the past but a rollercoaster nonetheless. I fell madly in love, made some mistakes, got my heart broken, started my business, made more mistakes, lost my sister, got married again, made more mistakes, became a mother, made even more mistakes, lost my father, marriage broke up.

So I realised I needed some tools, some ways to help me deal with these challenges now that I'd effectively said, 'Bring it on!' I attended workshops, delved into ancient texts, spoke to like-minded people, meditated, journalled and explored, and so began to discover ways of doing The Real Work *and* coming out the other side with glowing, vibrant energy!

Case Study

'What next?' A client said to me today. Nick had completely burned out at work. He'd been off work for two months and saw me for a few sessions during this time. His was a pretty straightforward case of cleaning up energy and helping him to get some decent sleep. He was back at work and feeling optimistic. He had absolutely no regrets about what had happened and felt the whole experience had taught him so much. He now wanted to understand how to stop what had happened from happening again – he'd certainly learnt about how to physically look after himself better but he had a hunch that there was some deeper work that needed to happen. In particular, why he had a tendency to push himself so hard to the exclusion of everything else. He was ready for The Real Work.

None of this was done from a mountaintop or ashram (if only) but from within the thick of life with all of its trials and tribulations. Over time, life started to feel more like an adventure rather than a battleground. I was growing stronger and more resilient and I was experiencing more joy and happiness.

Then, exactly the same magic happened as had with my sleep work; as I worked on my life challenges and spiritual growth, so more opportunities started coming up for me to teach others what I was learning. I know that part of this was due to the Fast Asleep, Wide Awake formula at work – solving people's sleep and energy problems was leading them towards doing The Real Work in a natural trajectory. But I'm convinced that something weird and wonderful was also at play and it was as if I was being given an opportunity to work even more deeply with people – with their lives and their consciousness – and to teach from my own experience.

Again, it was the same process of working with many people and discovering that, yes, I could help them sleep and break the fatigue cycle but they then needed deeper tools and techniques because the conversation had changed. They were no longer in SURVIVAL mode and wanting to know how to sleep or how to stop feeling more exhausted. They were asking different questions and wanting different answers.

- 'I can see why I've been so unhappy, but what does happiness mean? How do I find it? How do I feel passion again?'
- 'How do I truly feel safe?'
- 'What is it that I really want to do with my life? What is my life purpose?'
- 'I've achieved so much in life but why can't I celebrate my success? Why am I so hard on myself?'
- 'There's so much uncertainty in my life right now. How do I work out what to do next?'
- 'How do I overcome my fears?'

As I said previously, it took me at least a couple of decades to find answers to these questions – and I'm still learning – but the good news is that it really doesn't have to take that long, as the Energy for Life Programme can *fast track the route*. The tools you'll learn in the next chapter will help you to navigate The Real Work and guide you to:

- Find a constant source of inner strength and calm, even in chaos.
- Identify and create an internal guidance system that will keep you on track while on The Real Work journey.
- Find self-acceptance and self-love.
- Build strong supports so you're not doing this on your own.
- Manage difficult feelings as they arise.
- Learn how to accept that which is beyond your control.
- Maintain your body in a resourceful and healing state so that you can continue to do The Real Work with vibrant energy.
- Establish good routines and rhythms so that you're not tempted to give up.
- Find the gem or meaning so that you don't stay stuck.

With these tools you will be able to deal with whatever was stopping you sleeping and draining your energy in the first place and receive the biggest reward of all – extraordinary energy.

The Glow

Throughout this book I've been promising you vibrant, extraordinary energy and this is what you start to get when you get to this stage. This is one of the greatest rewards for all your efforts. Recently I asked a dear friend who's been going through some health and relationship problems how she's feeling. She replied, 'I've got a spring in my step.' She's now dealing with things head on. Her problems are far from resolved but she's found something – a place within – from which she can deal with her situation more resourcefully. I can spot this shift in someone from a long way off – be it their active energy, an aura of peace and calm, a glow.

Earlier, I talked about how the chakras – our energy and power centres – can become blocked with old stagnant energy when we avoid dealing with our problems and this can eventually cause imbalances and disease (*see page 75*). As you begin to do The Real Work, you begin to unblock the chakras – and you will start to glow.

I see this all the time with my clients – they literally start to exude energy, and you can see it in their eyes. For example, I saw it in a client who came to see me recently. Her husband had committed suicide, leaving her with young children and a pile of financial worries, but despite all of this she had the glow. She was finding a way forward, challenging herself and making courageous choices. And another client plucked up the courage to leave her job in order to start a business that she felt passionately about. She was taking huge risks and, at one stage, even had to declare bankruptcy. She undoubtedly had many low points along the way but every time I saw her I could see glimpses of her 'glow' – even through the tears. Finally, she has landed on her feet and her business is taking off at a breakneck speed.

This is not something I can explain or describe in scientific terms, but it really is a glow. When I returned from Australia, the reality of my situation and all the big changes I was going to be making hit home. At times it was scary and overwhelming but so many people said to me, 'You look so well. You're glowing!'

There is something else that you can expect too, and that is you will discover a place within you, a refuge, a safe place from which you can start to live your life. Innumerable times clients have told me (and I've experienced this too) that once they've made this shift from survival to sustainable energy they discover something within themselves, which completely changes the way they make choices. They're no longer pulled this way and that by whatever is going on 'out there' but are deeply and wisely guided by something that lies deep within. Perhaps it's best described in the words that a client used recently: 'It's not God. But a connection to something bigger than all of the stuff I was fixating on and worrying about before. And it's within me.'

What Is the Place Within?

Neuroscientists have been asking this question for decades and in fact the quest to find a physical, brain-located source of religious and spiritual experience has even given birth to the science of 'neurotheology'. One of the main researchers in this field, V.S. Ramachandran, questions in his book *Phantoms in the Brain* whether there is 'some sort of circuitry that is actually specialised for religious experience? Is there a "God Module" in our heads? And if such a circuit exists, where did it come from?'

Whatever 'it' is – call it Ramachandran's 'God Spot' or even God, the Divine source, or a Higher Self, or inner strength – does it really matter how we label it? I can say with conviction that once you've found this place your life will become more peaceful and less of a struggle. And even though at times you'll find yourself right back in the same mulchy situations, making the same old mistakes, each time you grow wiser and stronger and notice that each time it gets easier because you have this safe, inner refuge to come back to. Karen Armstrong describes this journey in *The Spiral Staircase* thus: 'And as I go up, step by step, I am turning, again, round and round, apparently covering little ground, but climbing upwards, I hope towards the light.'

When you turn the page, the very first tool you will come to – I call it 'coming home' – will show you, in immensely practical terms (always my trademark) how to begin to find this place within yourself and how, once you have found it, you can strengthen the connection with it. How you choose to work with the Energy for Life Programme is entirely up to you but I do recommend starting with this first exercise, as it sets the stage and prepares you to go deeper with the other exercises. An open and curious mind is also a good starting point.

Chapter 11

The Energy for Life Programme

'The good life is one inspired by love and guided by knowledge.'

Bertrand Russell

The Energy for Life Programme contains what I have come to see as the spiritual tools that we can use for living life with amazing energy, sleeping deeply, and evolving and growing as human beings. I discovered them by chance as I sought to create safety and stability in my own life, but I know that I cannot claim that they are unique to me. Rather, I would describe them as coming from an ancient timeless wisdom that we've always had access to but have perhaps forgotten in this noisy, busy world we live in today. I hope you enjoy using them.

Come Home Regularly

Life can be chaotic and uncertain. There's so much choice these days, and knowing what to do in the moment can, at times, feel ridiculously overwhelming. Even buying a cup of coffee can feel choice-laden and confusing. Hardly surprising then that at the end of the day sleep can feel so noisy, wired and nightmarish.

This tool is about finding stillness so that you can find your answers, renew your energy and smooth out the noise. It is vital to you being able to self-diagnose and listen to your body more deeply. I call this 'coming home' because this is the familiar place that we return to in order to renew ourselves, gather our energy before we move forward to action. It is the place we must go to if we are to sleep purely and deeply. Home is also coming back into the body, away from thought and constant mental chatter. As John O'Donohue says in *Anam Cara*: 'The body is your only home.'

What happens when we become still is that we begin to listen to ourselves. By this I mean we quieten down so that we can hear. You may be shocked by the noisiness of your mind when you first start doing this, but the more you do it, the easier it will become to allow the noise to happen and to just observe it.

I really believe that one of the biggest reasons that I'm seeing more young people at my clinic with panic attacks is because they've lost the ability to do this. So they only meet themselves when that inner voice starts yelling at them – and by then it feels panicky and scary. If we allow ourselves to encounter our noisy minds regularly during the day, then it becomes less scary and overwhelming at night when the lights are out.

You might want to sign up for a meditation or mindfulness course or check out the Headspace website for guided mindfulness programmes (www.headspace.com). However, many people embark on such programmes and then abandon them when life gets busy and stressful, ironically the times when they really need to be using such techniques. I am a great believer in finding practical and simple ways of making this principle work for you in simple, doable ways so that it becomes second nature and you use it *especially* when life is challenging.

Here are some practical ways of coming home:

1. **First thing:** The most powerful time to come home is first thing in the morning. What is your first choice of the day? Do you roll over and press the snooze button? Grab your phone and start checking your emails and messages? Do you worry about what lies ahead in the day? The way you start your day has a powerful knock-on effect on the rest of your day – as does the way you end your day, as we explored earlier. Start your day by meeting yourself using the 'noticing three exhalations' exercise (*see page 140*) even while lying in bed.

2. **Look deeply at yourself:** When you visit the bathroom, look in the mirror into your eyes while washing your hands. Let go of thinking about what you were doing before or what you are going to do next. Think of this practice as 'washing off' whatever you have just dealt with so that you can move on to the next part of your life. Look deeply into your eyes, breathe deeply and come back to yourself.

3. **Ground yourself:** As you go through your day make a point every now and then of feeling your feet on the ground, as you learnt to do in the 'grounding and rooting' exercise (*see page 153*). Even doing this for a minute or two can create a pocket of peace in a stressful day. Do this especially when your day is chaotic and demanding. Punctuate your day with several moments like this.

4. **Find silence:** Sit in silence for a minute. Turn off the TV or radio. Put down your phone. Stop talking. Be quiet and close your eyes. You might want to experiment with doing this first thing in the morning, last thing at night and then two or

three times during the day. You don't have to put hours of time aside. A minute here or there while standing in line, doing the dishes, chopping the onions, before you open up your inbox.

You may find, when you start to experience the benefits of such quiet time, that you become more creative about how you eke out such moments even in a busy, buzzy environment.

Nathan, a lawyer, would find an empty meeting room where he could just sit and breathe for a few minutes. Paul, a city banker, would sit quietly on a pew in a church and close his eyes. Initially he'd started doing this because he was so tired and it was his way of seeking out some mid-afternoon rest whenever he could. But soon he began to feel that these 10 minutes or so were such a bolster for his spirits and that when he returned to the office somehow things just didn't seem so stressful.

> **Allow yourself time to do nothing and you'll come to realise that doing nothing is actually doing something.**

Case Study

Sally, a busy mother of three children, would sit quietly in her car before school pick-up. Previously she'd sit listening mindlessly to whatever was on the radio while playing with her phone. Choosing to sit in silence even for a few minutes before collecting her children from school made such a difference to the way she was able to relate to them when they started making demands on her. And she was amazed that she hardly ever needed to shout any more. Eventually she began to find that she'd become very adept at tuning out and tuning in, even when she was surrounded by noise. Once she'd found that place within her she realised that she could choose to go there even when she was in a busy grocery store.

Allow yourself to be with silence and you'll notice that silence is a sound you've been craving for quite some time. Daydream or sit and wonder (wondering is a powerful tool). Whether you choose to join a meditation or mindfulness class, take up a quiet form of yoga, tai chi or chi kung, or simply sit with a sketchbook and draw or start keeping a journal, research shows that spending time in quiet contemplation or meditation offers a hosts of benefits to our well-being, including boosting health, happiness, brain and productivity.[28]

You don't have to make a big song and dance about doing this or sit cross-legged for hours in the lotus position – your coming home might be walking the dog or getting your hands into the soil while gardening. In short, it is whatever is your version of coming home.

> You really don't need props or any special location. This is simply about learning how to tune out distraction.

After you've been doing this for a while you will notice that you start coming home naturally without needing to consciously make time to do it. Then you can expect some positive changes in your life. At the very least, you will notice that you feel less busy and stressed and more able to respond to life's challenges rather than reacting to them. You will most likely find that your sleep improves too and feels less scratchy and noisy. Your relationship with yourself, your self-awareness, becomes more honed and you may begin to question the choices you've been making and whether they really are the most helpful ones for you. Patterns in your relationships will take on a new light as you start to see how you have been influencing them.

Invariably, as we find our rituals and rhythms for turning inwards, we begin to develop a stronger connection to ourselves and a bigger connection to life itself, that many refer to as the Divine or consciousness (*see page 76*). And from this, if we nurture it and allow this connection to build, comes trust and faith. This is when we truly start to build a strong core and backbone for dealing with life. This is when we can sleep despite the inevitable challenges we face in life.

Commit to using at least one of these practices every day for the next three weeks and just notice how your energy feels.

Find Your 'Why?'

So many people struggle to get out of bed in the morning and start their day with energy. We all need a reason to get out of bed in the morning. When you find your 'why?' it focuses your energy – you have a purpose for your energy and it is less likely to feel splintered – so this tool is about finding that reason, your 'why?'

Take Karen, a young woman in my morning patient group, who complained that she just couldn't get out of bed in the morning and that she tended to sleep for hours during the day too. In fact, she was escaping into sleep. Her 'why?' was that she was so tired all the time.

Why?
She was going to bed too late, wasn't eating breakfast, and living on caffeine, sugary snacks and drinks. All the stuff you've read about in the first part of this book.

Why?
It was easy. She knew that the way she was running her body wasn't healthy but she couldn't stop doing it.

Why?
She couldn't be bothered to change.

Why?
What was the point? She hated what she was doing with her life anyway.

But when Karen found her why she plucked up courage to ask for a move within the company. She ended up relocating to another branch whose offices were in a quieter, more rural part of the country (nature was important to her) and following more of her creative interests. She wrote to tell me that most days she woke up looking forward to the day ahead.

We all need a reason to get out of bed in the morning. Of course, there will be times when we settle for the easy option. We've all done the jobs where we've had to tread water for a time, just to pay the bills, but the time comes when meaning is important. Otherwise our life force gets stuck, we become sick and can't sleep or we oversleep, as in Karen's case.

This tool probably underpins everything you've read in this book so far. It's the 'why?' behind it all.

- Why would you bother taking time out to breathe deeply or meditate?
- Why would you bother to count your blessings? In fact, why exercise or eat healthily?

Superficial motivations never drive lasting behaviour change. Which is the reason why most diets don't work and people waste money on gym memberships.

In order to make truly lasting changes, we need to find our deeper motivations and drives so that doing what we set out to do becomes so imperative that it overrides the pain of the unfamiliar. When we go deeper and work out what we truly care about and value in life, then we are more likely to do what is necessary. We become laser focused about what we need to do.

We are constantly changing – apparently the entire human body, however many trillions of cells, is completely renewed every seven years. But if we don't pay attention we can end up running on the same old script and thinking the same old things are important to us without even realising that we are heading in the wrong direction. If we're rushing around at top speed we don't notice, even though the body tries to tell us – it tries to slow us down, we get aches and pains, mystery illnesses, sleeplessness – anything to make us slow down and pay attention.

For example, five years ago I gave up marathon running because I realised my values had changed. I had changed. I paid attention and discovered that running marathons was no longer the thing for me. And why? Like many parents, I have a value around being a good mother. For me, this means spending quality time with my daughter, having the energy to play with her, listen to her, even if I've had a stressful day. I noticed that, as I got older, marathon training was affecting my ability to do these things wholeheartedly (because I was tired!).

Your values are your 'sat nav' coordinates guiding the choices you make in life.

When we know what is important to us in life, it guides our behaviours and choices. It's a bit like plugging the coordinates into a sat nav and then letting it guide us in the right direction. Knowing what we care about and value is our inner sat nav, but if you've never taken the time to think about such things you end up throwing your energy around in a dissipated and scattered fashion and risk missing out on the things that matter the most.

Take the practical example of eating breakfast – the habit that so many people struggle with. When we know what is important to us in life then uncomfortable choices become effortless and non-negotiable.

Now it's over to you …

Do you know what you care about? Truly care about?

Identifying Your Values

My friend Tracy Skyrme, co-owner of The Work Playground, designed the following exercises. She works with hard-nosed business professionals – many of whom have lost their way – and shows them how to reconnect with their value system so that they can get their lives back on track. The exercises are simple and even fun, but they can very effectively take you to the core of your values and how you want to live your life. You might choose to do just one of the exercises or all of them, if you have the time – they all take you to the same place.

Write a Story about Your 'Ideal Day'

This is not an exceptional or special day, just how you would like your daily life to be. Use as much detail as you can by including how you feel, what's important and why, who would be with you and what makes the day ideal. Really daydream and use your imagination. Look for themes throughout your ideal day – feelings, thoughts, actions, things that come up more than once, as these are likely to be connected to your values, or whatever makes sense for you.

Make a Collage

Get some magazines, glue and some paper – you can do this as a family, with your partner or on your own. Cut out images, words and phrases that stand out for you. Pictures that make you smile, which touch your heart or connect with you – words, colours, people, animals and so on. Stick them onto a large piece of paper – in whatever way works for you. What do you notice about your collage? What does it tell you about what is important to you?

Write a Dating Profile

Imagine you are writing a dating profile. What would you say about yourself? What is important to you? What can you not live without? What do you stand for? What will you fight for? What makes you happy? What makes you sad? Finally distil the description of yourself into three words.

Find What's Important

Think of a place in the world that you love – close your eyes and imagine that place. It could be close to home or far away – use all your senses to picture that place in your mind. What can you see, hear, smell, taste, touch? Open your eyes and use three words to describe that place. Write the words down using the sentence, 'I am [*insert your three words*].' How are these words important to you? What do they show about what is important to you and what makes you who you are?

Identify Your Characteristics

This is a great one for families. Each person identifies an animal they are like. Draw that animal or find a picture in a magazine. Describe how you are like that animal – talk to each other about the characteristics you have described. How does the person you are talking to recognise that in you? How do they know you are like that? What do they see or experience? Swap partners so you can share your animals and how it is like you.

> Write a few of the key words, your personal sat nav coordinates which you've discovered from using the above exercise/s, on a sticky note and place it where you can see it often. Allow those words to start guiding your behaviour.

These exercises will take you very quickly to the core of your values and how you want to live your life. You may find that you start to make small changes but with greater conviction and then they become habit as your internal dialogue changes from, 'I should do x, y or z' to 'I'm doing this because …'

When you bring your values into your conscious mind, you may find that when you start making choices based on your value system your energy starts to shift in a very positive direction.

Self-love

Many of the patients who end up at my sleep clinic are perfectionists, as are a large percentage of those attending the corporate auditoriums where I speak. Typically, these people drive themselves hard, finding it impossible to ask for help or to say 'no'. They are totally unable to put themselves and their needs first and, by the time they arrive at the clinic, are often completely disconnected from their body and its needs.

Their relationship with control is strong and so they are usually successful (at least up until the point of breakdown) and typically work for high-performance organisations. They run on fear-driven imperatives – have-to-dos, should-dos, must-dos. (I call the latter 'musterbation' and I'm deliberately being crude to make a point and hopefully it will stick in your mind.)

Every time you find yourself 'musterbating', stop and check yourself.

Typically perfectionists find it hard to relax and feel guilty about doing so. They find it hard to stay in the present; they live in and for the future (catastrophising) – forever working to be in control – or in the past (worrying and ruminating). Psychologists would say their locus of control is external – when everything out there is completely okay then I'll be okay. This, of course, is madness because it's never going to be completely okay out there. These are the ones who carry tightness in their neck and shoulders and grind their teeth at night. They tend to be prone to chronic fatigue and burnout. And of course they can't sleep.

Can you relate to this?

What really lies at the core of this is your relationship with yourself. And what really lies at the core of this perfectionism is a lack of self-love. If you never bother to nurture yourself then you'll be less likely to make healthy choices such as eating breakfast, taking a lunch break, accepting the support of others, or even accepting the support of your mattress and sleep.

I Am Enough

This simple exercise can shift your mind-set from 'not feeling good enough' to 'being enough' if you use it enough times, and it's simply this:

1. Look at yourself in the mirror and say the words, 'I am enough.'
2. Look into your eyes and say it with conviction, even if you don't believe it.
3. Say it first thing in the morning and remind yourself to say it throughout the day, before that presentation, while sitting in a traffic jam or waiting for a meeting to start.
4. Write the words 'I am enough' on a sticky note and attach it to your bathroom mirror.

This is called a positive affirmation (*see page 148*) and if done regularly – I recommend every morning for the next 21 days – it will start to change your relationship with yourself and the way you speak to yourself.

> If you want to take this exercise to the next level look at yourself in the mirror first thing in the morning and say the words 'I love you' too.

You may find this difficult to do at first and feel embarrassed by the idea of talking to yourself in a mirror, but really what have you got to lose? Amazing changes occur when you try these affirmations – from attracting more loving relationships to stepping out of your comfort zone and overcoming huge fears and blocks.

Case Study

Recently Arianna, a 16-year-old drama student, started using the 'I am enough' affirmation. Within two weeks she'd stopped having panic attacks and had been given the lead part in the school production. When she texted me her news she added, 'Think I'm ready to start telling myself "I love you" ☺.'

Quieten Your Inner Critic

The way you talk to yourself, your internal dialogue, has a powerful and measurable effect on how you feel and perform in daily life. Athletes are well aware of this, which is why they might work with a sports psychologist or coach to identify more powerful ways of speaking to themselves in order to perform at their best (*see page 148*).

The performance coach and author of *Ahead of the Game*, Jeremy Lazarus, coaches business and sports people and notes how, when tested, we are 'without exception' physically stronger when we think of a 'positive event' and use 'positive imagery and self-talk'.

Notice Your Voice

Become aware of how you speak to yourself. Does it energise you or make you feel deflated? Does it make you tense up or relaxed? Use the following exercise to help you start to notice the quality of your self-talk.

1. Say your name to yourself. Say it silently, sweetly and softly. How does it make you feel?
2. Now say it again silently but this time say it in a hard, barking voice, as if you're speaking to a badly behaved child.
3. Turn up the volume on this voice so it's really yelling at you. How does this make you feel?

You might be surprised to feel that the two voices immediately change your physical state and that the first voice helps you to soften and maybe even smile, while the second voice makes you tense and you might even find yourself holding your breath.

You may not be aware of it but your inner critic (or even several of them) may have spent many years creating tension in your mind and body, and it has not only served to exhaust you and stop you sleeping, but might also have stopped you from reaching your goals and taking risks.

The great thing about practices such as yoga, meditation and mindfulness or even the simple exercises I've described in this book – for example, the 'notice three exhalations' tool (*see page 140*) – is that they make you more aware of how you are talking to yourself. When you become aware, you can then decide whether to buy into your inner critic's voice or tell it where to go.

Become Aware of Your Inner Critic

The following three-step formula can help you notice when your inner critic is barking at you and whether it is something you want to listen to and act on.

1. **Become aware:** Notice how you are speaking to yourself and when you are using imperatives and how they are making you feel. You may notice guilt, worry, fear and even shame.
2. **Notice that it has a voice:** Is it a man or a woman? Over time you may notice that you have several voices and that they are related to specific situations. For example, I have a voice (that of a much feared biology teacher) that pops up when I sit down to write. Another voice when I'm in certain social situations where I feel I don't fit in well. This voice is the very young me who was very shy and self-effacing at school and who stammered a lot of the time (ironic given that much of my work now involves public speaking).
3. **Name your voice:** Give the voice a name that feels relevant. My writing voice is called Miss Trunchbull (from Roald Dahl's *Matilda*). She looks and sounds remarkably like my old biology teacher. When Miss Trunchbull pops up and tells me I can't write (usually every time I sit down at the keyboard) I tell her in no uncertain terms where to go. If I listened to this voice I'd never write, I'd go and do some housework or check my Facebook page or email – so many options.

By noticing this aspect of yourself, you become the observer of the voice. In becoming the observer, you begin to separate from it rather than believing its story. You can choose whether to act on the voice or to opt for a different, perhaps kinder, behaviour.

Case Study

I once had an extremely perfectionistic client who, along with not sleeping very well, kept falling over and spraining her ankles. An odd connection, you might think, but we realised that her accidents were due to her constant rushing around and fear of being late. This came from the voice that was constantly telling her to 'hurry up'. When she did the above exercise she realised that it was her father's voice. He was a strict disciplinarian who punished her for even being a few minutes late. Becoming aware of her inner critic helped her to break the pattern and slow down – and it was kinder on her ankles too.

If there's a particular voice or pattern that you want to work on, make an intention to be more aware of it for the next 21 days. Ask a close friend or family member to support you in doing this. Check in with yourself after this time and see if anything has changed.

Accepting Support

Nocturnal restlessness is often partly due to our inability to lean back and accept support in life. We're always holding on, unable to let go and trust. But once you start working on your inner critic's voice(s), you may notice that for a long time you've been trying to go it alone. It takes courage to acknowledge that we all need help and support. Reflect on the following questions to find where you, perhaps, need more support.

- How are you supporting yourself at the moment?
- What are you doing to give yourself the right type of energy to face whatever life is throwing at you?
- Who's on your side?
- Who can you laugh with?
- Who can you cry with?
- Who in your life will genuinely listen to you without interruption or trying to diagnose or fix things?

If there is someone in your life who can support you in this way then that relationship is a rare gem to be cherished, and we usually don't make these types of connections on social media, no matter how many 'likes' our last post attracted.

If you don't have support in your life, where can you find some? It might be a counsellor or therapist who can help to support you through difficult times. Support might also take the form of starting a meditation practice or going to the gym. It might be joining a singing or dancing club. Support is anything that helps you to let go of negative emotions, fills you up and nourishes you.

Be Open to Receiving Support

If you can't identify any true and reliable supports in your life then I invite you to use the following affirmation as often as you can: 'I am open to receiving support in my life.'

Just keep saying it to yourself over the following days and especially as you drift off to sleep and on waking. Write it down too and keep looking at it. And see what starts to happen. Remember the power of affirmations and mantras that I described earlier (*see page 148*) – they have the power to change your mind-set and using 'I am open to receiving support in my life' can help you be more open to finding the right person or activity to support you.

If you hit a tough spot, don't be afraid to ask, 'What do I need to help me get through this? Who can help me get through this?' Seek out people who can support you and mirror back to you, so that you can see more clearly where you are in life and what needs to be done next. Seek the support that will stop you reverting back to old, unhelpful patterns.

Use your intuition to guide your choices when looking for help.

Case Study

A client came to see me a while ago. Originally from Venezuela, she had spent much of the last 20 years bringing up her two children and living in different countries, as her husband's work took him around the world. She had a fixed smile on her face and actually made a point of saying, 'I smile a lot,' but there was a sad story behind her sleeplessness. She missed 'home' desperately and, in particular, her mother with whom she was very close. Over the last few years she'd had a number of serious health scares including two bouts of cancer. It was clear to me that she needed more support in her life but she told me that she found it hard to trust people, to show them how she was feeling, and consequently had very few close friends. Her father had told her many times when she was young that she was 'emotionally stupid'. She felt he hadn't really meant it but the words had stuck in her mind and prevented her from finding the support she needed.

If you feel it could be helpful to get extra help, take a look at the Resources section (*see page 247*) for a list of recommended practitioners, coaches and therapists who can support you on your journey.

Allow Your Feelings

Repressed feelings can make their appearance in your sleep, creating vivid dreams, nightmares and teeth grinding. Or they wake you in the early hours and stop you getting back to sleep. Recent Swedish studies of over 2,000 adults showed that people who didn't express their emotions were more likely to develop insomnia. The lead researcher, Markus Jansson-Fröjmark, explained that 'teaching people strategies for regulating emotions might help prevent new cases of insomnia to occur and decrease the risk of persistent insomnia'.[29]

Often we live too much in the mental realm and our emotions and feelings get neglected as a result. A lot of the time you might not even know how you are feeling.

**It takes courage to allow yourself
to feel.**

Case Study

Susan had a breakthrough when she realised that her comfort eating in the evenings, aside from affecting her sleep, was an attempt to distract herself from sadness. She had adopted this strategy following her mother's death when she was very young and subsequently tended to use comfort eating at the end of the day to avoid feeling uncomfortable feelings.

If we don't allow ourselves to acknowledge our feelings, where do they go? Often into our unconscious brain and our sleep. How are you feeling right now? Do you even know?

We are so good at protecting ourselves from feeling. We keep busy, medicate with alcohol and drugs, chocolate, exercise, sex, or anything that stops us feeling. We turn up the radio or the TV and tune out. But in the process we become deadened, heavy, exhausted, sleepless, and so also stop ourselves from feeling joy and happiness too because, as the poet Kahlil Gibran says, 'Your joy is your sorrow unmasked.'

When you allow yourself to feel what needs to be felt, you might be surprised that after the 'wave' passes you feel relieved, lighter, less overwhelmed and then maybe even optimistic and happy.

Recently, I've seen a number of young people at my clinic whose problems – nightmares and night terrors, panic attacks and even self-harming behaviours – can be linked to an inability to feel what needs to be felt. They might come from stable, supportive homes but what they lack is an ability to feel sadness, or rather an ability to *allow* themselves to feel sadness.

Susan Stiffelman is a family therapist and 'Parent Coach' who writes for the *Huffington Post*. In her book *Parenting with Presence* she calls this 'dry-eyed syndrome' in which a fear of feeling sadness causes emotions to be held in and repressed and then acted out in other ways (tantrums) or in physical imbalances. In my work, the point when my client cries usually signals the breakthrough.

> You may want to take a look at the Sedona Method[30] or a similar programme in which you can actually learn how to feel what you're feeling before it builds up to an unhealthy level and starts to create illness.

Now I want to offer you some exercises and techniques for dealing with emotions, which you might want to experiment with in small ways that feel safe for you. For example, when you are fearful before a presentation, angry with a fellow commuter or frustrated with your teenager.

Diving In

Use this exercise if you become aware of anxiety or sadness just before you go to bed so you avoid taking that energy into your sleep. The 'cutting the cords' exercise described in Chapter 9 (*see page 155*) is another effective way of disconnecting before sleep.

1. Get quiet. Breathe deeply and steadily into the feeling.
2. Can you identify the feeling? Is it anger or fear or sadness or something else?

3. Feel the feeling.
4. When you recognise it, say to yourself: 'I am angry [*or afraid, sad, scared, etc.*].'
5. Feel the feeling some more. Become the feeling by saying, 'I am anger' (or fear, sadness, etc.).
6. Do what you need to do to go with the wave of emotion: breathe more deeply into it, cry, howl or scream, if necessary. Initially you might feel a little numb, as if you're not feeling anything at all, or you may notice that the 'wave feeling' builds to a climax and then dissipates. Observe that you don't stay immersed in the feeling forever (this is a common fear and the main reason why we don't like to feel negative feelings).
7. Notice the lightness that comes afterwards.
8. To avoid holding on to the feelings unnecessarily, you'll now want to change your energy state by doing an activity that brings you back to yourself, for example:
    * Light a candle and meditate or focus on your breath for 5–10 minutes.
    * Wash your face, while looking into your eyes as you do – in order to come back to yourself.
    * Use the 'earthing, grounding and rooting' exercise (*see page 154*).
    * Go for a brisk walk or run.
    * Sit quietly outside in the fresh air for 5–10 minutes with a glass of water or cup of herbal tea.

The AAAAHHH Breath

Sometimes our feelings have so much energy that they need to be released. Talking sometimes just make things worse, as we get tied up in knots with complicated stories and justifications of why we're feeling this way.

For example, I often see people walking home from the train station at the end of the day and they look as though they are talking to themselves – and sometimes they actually are. I wonder if they are saying the things they couldn't say during the day. Or, after a frustrating conversation in which we couldn't say what we wanted to say, we might groan out loud with jaw clenched, holding in that AAAAHHH frustration. What we need is some sort of physical release.

As babies, we signalled and released pain by crying, making the sound, 'AAAAHHH'. We didn't try to construct words and stories because we couldn't – the stories and interpretations come as we grow older – so we simply released the sound 'AAAAHHH'.

The following technique is a simple way to release pent-up emotions but can also be helpful in stopping teeth grinding during the night – and so avoid dental bills.

1. Find a space away from everyone. Ideally you really want to be as private as possible because you're going to make some noise.
2. Gently hold your jaw between finger and thumb, allow your jaw to go slack and try to waggle it. Let some sound out at the same time. You may notice that your jaw is very tight, which indicates that you're holding your emotions in.
3. Now for the brave bit. Open your jaw as wide as you can without hurting yourself and say, 'AAAAAHHH'. Keep repeating it for 5 minutes, pausing between breaths. Allow yourself to release whatever sound comes instinctively – it might start as a gentle sigh but then build up to a thunderous bellow.

One of my clients drives to a field, parks her car and then lets out her AAAAHHH breath. Another client says she can't do this at home, as it would scare the kids, so she does it soundlessly in the shower and imagines a thick grey cloud leaving her mouth as she does it (a bit like the scene from the movie *The Green Mile*). Be creative and playful but don't underestimate the power of this technique.

Dumping the Bricks

Crying and laughing are also powerful ways of releasing energy and rebalancing your system. I used to be afraid of crying – so many people are – but now I'm proud to say, 'I love a good cry.' In my marathon running days I'd often have a good cry the day before the race and I'm convinced it made me faster. Our coach used to call this 'dumping the bricks'. A good cry frees and cleanses you. We can learn a lot about crying by observing how babies do it: they take a deep breath in and then – wait for it – they let rip and let the sound out on the out-breath without holding back. This is then followed by short, rapid inhalation sobs as they quieten down.

The next time you feel a wave of feeling come over you and an impulse to cry or laugh, notice your breathing and allow it to support you. Give yourself permission to cry like a child – this is not weakness.

It takes courage to feel the feelings and let go.

Practising Acceptance

Change is an inevitable part of life – we all know that. Nothing ever stays the same. Nature is a perfect reflection of this in its changing seasons, the waxing and waning moon, the cells of the body constantly renewing themselves, the life cycle of birth and death, and so on. But change can be scary and unsettling. We wake in the early hours, usually 2–4 a.m., tossing and turning. Everything seems so much worse in the dark, when all is quiet, and the unconscious mind is at its most creative so that the smallest of problems seem insurmountable.

Although we know that change is inevitable, the world is full of people trying to control and change the things they can't and not ignoring the things they can (usually because they're exhausted, fearful and/or not sleeping). We hold back and resist change and the body feels it. We feel it in our joints – ankles, knees, hips, back – as we resist change and so become hardened and inflexible.

Many of the clients that come to see me are initially in this hardened and inflexible state, which manifests as muscle tightness and/or back and joint pain, as well as exhaustion and sleeping issues. All they want is to learn how to sleep – nothing else – but it's usually evident that their sleeping issues are due to resisting change.

For example, take the man whose marriage is on the rocks after discovering his wife's infidelities. He doesn't want to think about it. All he wants to talk about is how exhausted he is and that he can't sleep. Understandably, he hasn't got the energy to do The Real Work and the way I see it is that it's not my place to interfere with the process. We clean up his energy and he starts getting some decent sleep and feels more invigorated so that by the third session he says, 'I'm going to see a therapist. I'm not sure what I want to do about my marriage yet but right now I need to work out who I am and what I want in life.'

It makes sense that we should embrace change. But how do we do that? We have to step into the unknown, and this can be scary.

One of the reasons I love climbing is that it teaches me to navigate uncertainty. If I stretch up for this hold will I reach it? And if I do, will I be able to maintain my grip or will I fall? Usually (but not always) I'm on a rope so it's a calculated risk, but it's still scary because our ego is primed to tell us not to trust, that we will fall and we won't survive.

I Wonder ...

All of the tools in this Energy for Life Programme can bring about a simple shift in mind-set to help you to embrace uncertainty with more courage. However, I'd like to offer you a simple but effective technique for dealing with matters that aren't in your control, simply by reframing them (*see page 150*). In other words, changing the language of how you think or speak about them.

Using the words 'I wonder ...' rather than 'I hope ...' seems such a small thing but it can create a huge shift in your mind-set, which is vital in softening your grip on life. The next time you're facing uncertainty, embrace change by asking:

- I wonder what will happen if the train doesn't turn up on time ...
- I wonder what will happen if I fail my exams ...
- I wonder what will happen if I don't get that house I want to buy ... (This is an excellent game to play when buying a house.)

And then the big scary stuff of life:

- I wonder what will happen if I lose my job ...
- I wonder what will happen if my relationship ends ...
- I wonder what will happen if he or she dies ...

It might sound virtually impossible to think this way if you're not used to it, but just be curious and experiment with it. For the next few days, every time you find yourself tightening up, jaws clenching, shoulders heading north, just stop and look at the situation you're trying to control and ask, 'How much control do I really have? Really?' Then use the following three-step letting-go exercise:

1. Be honest with yourself and then say, 'I wonder what will happen if ...'
2. Let it go by saying, 'I let go of this situation.'
3. Imagine a cord that is attached to the problem, which is going straight into your solar plexus. Take an imaginary pair of scissors, cut the cord and release it into an imaginary fire or actual candle flame while saying, 'I let go of this problem,' as you did in the 'cutting the cords' exercise (*see page 155*).

Even more powerful is to repeat the words, 'I let go and let God decide.'

**Trust that life is happening
for you and not to you.**

Flood Your Body with Legal Highs

Earlier I explained why sleeping tablets or other forms of medication are not the answer to your sleep problem (*see page 3*). They might offer some short-term respite but in the long term they can make the problem worse as they stop the body's own innate balancing processes from working naturally.

Our body has an incredible innate intelligence: trillions of cells working in harmony to produce hormones, neurotransmitters and other chemical messengers that regulate every physiological process in the body. You've read about melatonin, the sleep hormone, produced by the pineal gland (*see page 45*), but the body also produces another set of related hormones, which make us feel happy, joyful, safe, loving, peaceful, mellow, inspired, passionate – all those hormones that we produce when we're running in our sustainable or SAFETY energy system (*see page 44*). These hormones make us feel alive and motivated to move forward in life.

Serotonin regulates our mood and helps us to relax so it's vital in preparing the body to let go and allow the full effects of melatonin to kick in. Many of the patients I see are serotonin depleted and are on drugs – one of the most popular being Prozac – that help to prolong the action of whatever minuscule amounts of serotonin they are producing.

Then we have the neuropeptide hormone oxytocin, also called the 'love hormone' because we produce it in large measure when we fall in love. Can you remember that feeling when you fall in love – that slightly mad, euphoric feeling? It is produced in the brain and in the heart, and plays its part in optimising our health in so many different ways:

- strengthening the immune system
- inducing labour in pregnant women
- breast milk letdown from the mammary glands
- aiding digestion
- protecting the heart from disease
- reducing inflammation in the body

In fact I could fill this book with an account of the important actions of oxytocin. But for the purposes of what we are here to talk about – doing The Real Work and solving life's problems and thereby sleeping and living well – oxytocin is vital.

Oxytocin could also be called the 'trust hormone' because this is what it does – it enables us to build trusting relationships with others: the newborn baby trusts its mother, we trust in our relationships and business – and we trust life. And as I've said so many times before, in order to sleep we need to feel safe. So oxytocin is the ultimate 'safety' hormone and therefore the ultimate sleep-inducing aid.

The reason I'm telling you about these wonderful hormones is that, while life can be tough, nature has also given us the innate means to rise above the pain and not get stuck, and in the process heal the body naturally. We have millions of cells in the body that are primed and ready to produce these mood-enhancing hormones; all we have to do is to trigger them. All we have to do is make the choices that will activate these natural highs and flood our bodies with healing and lightness.

**We can choose to gravitate
(get stuck in the mulch of life) or
radiate (rise up out of the mulch
and acknowledge the good in life).**

But how? Here are a few surprisingly practical ways:

Count Your Blessings

Every Tuesday morning when I work with my patients at the psychiatric clinic we get to a point in the session when I ask them to think about anything that's happened in their day so far that they are grateful for. It's usually around 10 a.m. so they often start off the exercise thinking they'll be hard pushed to find anything at all (very rarely has anyone never found anything – not even the most depressed patients).

**Everyone can find at least two
things that they are thankful for.**

There are myriad studies in the field of positive psychology and psychoneuroimmunology (PNI) that show that feeling grateful is good for your health.[31,32] Robert Emmons, one of the world's leading experts on the science of gratitude and co-author of *The Psychology of Gratitude*, says that being grateful boosts our immune system and physical health, it helps us to be more present and less worried about the future or depressed about the past, it blocks negative, toxic emotions, boosts your self-esteem and self-worth, makes us stress resistant and, if you hadn't guessed already, it helps us sleep.

We can so easily become consumed and overwhelmed by everyday stresses and responsibilities. Regularly practising gratitude isn't about pretending that life is perfect but acknowledging that we are blessed – if we are prepared to notice it. What I love about the 'notice three exhalations' exercise (*see page 140*) is that when we stop reacting to life, when we slow down and find that gap between the stimulus and response (*see page 142*), we start to notice. All of the small things – a supportive text message from a friend, your pet turning up to be stroked at just the right moment, a hot cup of tea, a seat on the train during the rush hour – when noticed and acknowledged gratefully these small gifts can have a powerful effect on your mind and body. What's more, research from the HeartMath Institute shows that heart rate variability – a good indicator of cardiac risk – is improved with gratitude exercises.[33]

Easy Practices for Cultivating Gratitude

1. Sit back, relax and take a deep breath. Now start to think about what you love, or even like, about the situation you're in right now. Look hard if you need to. What is good about where you are right now?
2. Have you been able to find anything positive about the situation you're in right now? Even the smallest thing?
3. Can you go a bit deeper and find a few more things? Can you challenge yourself to find as many small positive things about your situation as possible?
4. Having found something (or hopefully a few things), feel how this makes you feel. Breathe deeply into your heart, feeling gratitude for the situation or the person you're

thinking of. Breathe deeply and think about what you like or love about this situation.

5. Notice how you feel in your body. Is there a softening or slight relaxing? Have you let go slightly? What is your mood like now? Do you feel even a touch lighter? This is what I mean by 'radiating'. We become expansive, lifted up and out, even if momentarily, from life's difficulties.

The chances are, if you are reading this book, that you've had food today or will do at some point, you have a roof over your head, somewhere to sleep tonight. Maybe you've been able to have a hot shower or bath and put on clean clothes. Doing this exercise reminds us that we are blessed but we can so easily forget.

You might also like to try one or more of the following ideas:

• Keep a gratitude journal and make it a regular daily practice to write down a few things that have happened in your day for which you are grateful.

• Write a letter to someone who has positively influenced your life. Read it to them out loud or send it to them.

• Write a letter to someone who has challenged you in your life. Dig deep and think of all the reasons why you are grateful to them and what they have taught you (even inadvertently). You don't necessarily have to share this letter with them – this challenging exercise is purely for your benefit.

My dear friend and colleague, Gosia Gorna, teaches cancer patients gratitude exercises and meditation and says the difference it makes to their demeanour, ability to cope with discomfort and wellbeing is quite remarkable. When I recently went through my separation I downloaded a gratitude meditation from her website (www.gosiagorna.com) and listening to it at night helped me feel so peaceful and safe that I slept well.

Express Your Emotions

You've already heard from me on the importance of expressing your emotions (*see page 60*). In a nutshell, expressing yourself in a constructive way can boost levels of oxytocin. Repressing, on the other hand, suppresses oxytocin levels.

Acts of Kindness

Feeling grateful and counting your blessings is good for you and can even change the way your brain is wired (*see page 207*). Paying it forward – when you repay a good deed, not to the one who did it but to others – is even more powerful and expansive. According to David Hamilton in his book *Why Kindness Is Good for You*, kindness measurably changes the structure of your brain and causes the oxytocin-secreting cells in the heart and brain to rev up.

Acts of kindness don't have to mean grand gestures or giving expensive gifts and can be as simple as putting a few coins in a charity box or checking in on an elderly neighbour. If you want some ideas how you could give more then there are a number of websites, such as www.actionforhappiness. org, where you can find ideas for how you can help others in small ways that can make all the difference.

If you make the decision to practise acts of kindness, you will find that it soon becomes second nature. The heart chakra opens (*see page 78*) and our energy lifts and so we attract even more positive energy into our lives. Our health changes for the better and, of course, we sleep more peacefully. The strange thing I've noticed is that life starts to become more playful and less stress-laden too.

Feeling Good

Laughing, playing and dancing or simply watching your favourite comedy show bolsters levels of immunity-boosting immunoglobulin, natural killer cells and T-cells.[34] Studies also show that hugging – not just a cursory hug but real heart-to-heart hugging for at least a few minutes – increases oxytocin levels.[35]

Other practical ways to boost your oxytocin levels include massage, prayer, thinking about someone you love and sending them love, looking at a photograph of someone you love, stroking your pet and even lovingly looking after a houseplant.

Any sense of true connection produces oxytocin.

Enjoy the Commute

If, like me, you sometimes commute in a busy city, you will be familiar with the energy-sapping stress of it. I live a mere 21 kilometres (13 miles) from Central London but I have to allow at least 2 hours to get to my destination on time. That's 4 hours out of my day! After more than 20 years of doing this, I've come to see commuting as an opportunity to bathe in oxytocin, and here follow a few tricks for a restful commute – most of which can be done whether or not you get a seat:

- Avoid obsessively looking at your electronic devices.
- Avoid the free newspapers, which are invariably filled with doom and gloom.
- Read or listen to something uplifting.
- Meditate, even for just 5–10 minutes.
- Think of a beautiful place you've been to or a time when you felt at peace, relaxed and inspired.
- Think of someone you love and pray for him or her.
- Smile at your fellow commuters or dare to talk to them.
- Offer someone your seat.
- Pray for your loved ones, your fellow commuters or the world.
- Count your blessings.
- Remember what you care about.

Too many people lose sight of what gives them joy and start looking for it in all the wrong places – they live for their holidays or overindulge in retail therapy and so on. I believe that every day, and throughout the day, we should remind ourselves what we care about and make sure that we get a small injection of spiritual energy by connecting to these things – even in small measure. Don't wait for your weekends or your holidays or when you retire – by then it might be too late.

Nourishing what you care about gives you regular injections of spiritual energy.

One way to start bringing more of what you care about back into your life is to simply make a pact with yourself to start doing more of what you care about TODAY. Listen to a piece of music. Hug your child, but for longer than you normally would (remember the oxytocin effect). Switch your phone off on the way home from work and daydream or think about someone you love. Spend half an hour browsing in a bookshop and reading the first pages of a few books and see what captures your imagination. Or look at nature as you walk home, smell the air, look at the sky, notice the trees and birds, breathe deeply and come back into your body.

So many of us spend most of our time in workspaces that don't inspire us or make us feel happy, and so suppress the release of our natural mood-inducing hormones. Not surprisingly, we end up feeling depressed and dispirited and disconnected from what we truly care about.

To combat any negative effects and boost your serotonin production, surround your workspace with visual reminders of what you care about – pictures of your family, affirmations, poems, places you've visited, objects that mean something to you.

> If you hot-desk then travel light: take two or three items around with you, so that you always have reminders of the things that bring you joy.

I visit a lot of different offices and always have with me my moleskin notebook at the back of which I have my 'connectors' – a picture of my late father, a drawing my daughter made for me when she was three years old and an inspiring poem.

An important message here is don't forget what you care about. Regularly remind every cell of your body what truly matters to you.

You may have to give up something in order to make time for what you truly care about. This might mean weeding out some of the biggest time-wasters and energy drainers such as:

- Obsessively reading or watching the news.
- Surfing the Internet (have you noticed how quickly the time goes?).
- Checking your social media feeds and emails.
- Surfing TV channels or watching endless episodes of your current favourite box sets (occasionally enjoyable but not every night or into the early hours).
- Mindlessly doing all of the last three at the same time.

Making time for what truly matters is like adding that small pinch of nutmeg to your carrot cake – a small but vital amount of something that will enhance the taste and flavour. Life loses its special taste and flavour when we neglect what we truly care about. Just a small pinch … that's all you need. These days, with our busy lives, every 'yes' is a 'no' to something else. Do you know what you're saying 'no' to? And do you really want to?

Start on the Right Foot

Many times through this book I have recommended that you try a technique first thing in the morning. The way you start your day has a powerful impact on how the rest of the day unfolds and therefore how you sleep at night. When I began to change my morning routine, life itself began to change. It's all too easy to start the day bemoaning or dreading the day ahead or at the mercy of what's in your inbox or diary – I know because I used to do this too. Just a few seconds into the day and our energy is already being projected out there. So we begin the day in a state of fear and worry, amygdala fired up and adrenaline pumping through our veins. And this, of course, affects our appetite ... and so it goes on.

What if you started your day differently, and what would this look like? What if you started by drawing your energy in? Meeting yourself before you go out? This needn't even take many minutes out of your day – just a brief pause, even a few seconds, to gather yourself before you move to action.

The two most powerful words to start (and end) your day with are THANK YOU.

Even if you haven't slept that well, you thank your bed and your pillow. You thank God or yourself. You give thanks for all of the blessings in your life. Be creative but be grateful. And then notice the difference it makes to your day. Life is always going to present hurdles but at least if you start on the right foot you can meet them with a balanced and grounded stance. Here are a few more suggestions for how to start your day:

- With a smile - especially if you don't feel like smiling or if you're facing something that you're dreading.
- With 10–20 minutes of meditation, breath exercises, chi kung or yoga.
- Say, 'I love and approve of myself,' several times.
- Ground yourself - especially if you've got a hectic day ahead. Even while you're lying in bed imagine roots growing out of your feet and down into the ground all the way to the centre of the Earth. Breathe deeply through these roots and imagine them growing stronger and more grounding with each breath. Alternatively, do this while standing and really feel the ground beneath your feet.
- Repeat positive affirmations or prayers.

Look for the Meaning

Now I want to share with you the Ultimate Tool in the Energy for Life Programme. You will know when you are ready to use it.

When we find the true meaning of our suffering – the reason for our tiredness and sleepless nights – everything shifts: our energy, the way we sleep, our health and our perspective on life.

I'm often amazed at how much happened when I had my moment of awakening – so many realisations: that I was safe, that I wasn't alone, that I was being guided and protected, that I was surrounded and filled with a presence – call it grace or love – and that my suffering had meaning. I realised that I had been in a state of imbalance and *dis*-ease and every cell in my body had been trying to tell me something all along but I hadn't been listening. When I started listening – truly listening and understanding – I found the true meaning and I began to heal. Dr Kim Jobst, a medical doctor and integrated medicine physician, says, 'We need to see that, because disease is a manifestation of health, we can work with disease processes, gain understanding from them, and so use their energies to facilitate the healing responses that they invoke de facto.'[36]

Many of the people I've worked with have come to see that their sleep problem was a blessing in disguise and that without it they wouldn't have gone on to transform their lives in the way they did.

Case Study

One of my best friends in South Africa has battled with breast cancer for many years and ended up having radical surgery and secondary diabetic issues. Last week she sent me a message saying, 'I wouldn't take the terrible experiences back for anything in the world. I am in the light now and blessed for it.' She has been cancer-free for two years and I see her pictures on Facebook as she climbs mountains, kayaks, and runs 10k races with her husband and son. She glows with vibrant energy.

So what is the true meaning of your sleeplessness?

- What did you learn from it?
- What gifts did it bring?
- Has paying attention to it changed your life?
- What does it mean?

For example, did it mean that you started writing again? You and your partner sat down and committed to working on your relationship? Did you finally gather your courage and leave your job? Did you simply realise that life didn't have to be such a struggle and have you started letting go?

Where has the journey taken you and did you find the hidden gem?

Pay Attention and Start Noticing Synchronicities

When you start doing The Real Work you may begin to notice that life really starts to happen for you. Perhaps the right person or contact turns up at exactly the right moment. That encouraging text message pings into your phone just when you need it. Something that you might have thought would be a disaster turns out to be a blessing.

After my life-changing moment in Australia, I began to notice that 'coincidences' or, rather, synchronicities were taking place in my life all the time. It was as if I was being constantly guided and helped. I could describe many examples, but perhaps the moment that stands out was on 7 July 2005 when there was a terrorist attack on the London transport system. I was getting ready for a presentation in the City but my daughter, who was very young at the time, was ill so

I decided to stay at home – had I not I would have been trav-elling on the Underground just at the time when the bombs went off ...

As you become more attuned to yourself and your energy, pay attention to the seeming coincidences in your life and you will begin to see the patterns more and more often. But you do have to pay attention, as so often we don't notice them.

I love that scene from the film *Bruce Almighty* in which Jim Carrey is driving along the highway at top speed in a state of rage, bemoaning his life and shouting, 'God give me a sign!' All around him big signs are flashing 'SLOW DOWN, SLOW DOWN'. But he doesn't notice them.

Slow down and notice ... and you will find that it's so much easier to let go.

Chapter 12

Let the Magic Unfold

'Everybody's life has these moments, where one thing leads to another. Some are big and obvious and some are small and seemingly insignificant.'

Peter Jackson

I am now going to share three longer case studies with you. Not only do I want to demonstrate the programmes in action and show you how they work longer term, but also what can happen when you start to plug into your life force. Our natural energy is abundant, vibrant and transformational and we cannot stay stuck – as the following three stories indicate. These case studies are entirely true although the names and some of the personal details have been changed to hide the clients' identities.

Case Study 1: Finding True Purpose and Meaning

First Session

James, a 27-year-old personal trainer, came to see me over two years ago. In general, he was fit and healthy and a competitive weightlifter, however, he was experiencing several nightmares every night and at least two of them were night terrors. He was tired and desperate for help. The migraines he'd suffered as a child had returned and had worsened in the last six weeks. James occasionally experienced panic attacks while travelling or in crowded areas and had sought help for this in the past. Although his business was going well, there were several areas of his life that weren't: his relationships with his long-distance girlfriend and flatmates were strained, and he didn't find it easy to relax in the evenings – often playing computer games late into the evening to wind down.

James grew up in Guernsey and had happy childhood memories. He moved to London when he was 18. Although he enjoyed the professional success the move brought, he missed the peace and tranquillity of his family home. He loved being in nature but lately was spending less time doing so. He noticed that his sleep problems were starting to affect his energy levels and quality of life, and described feeling a general unhappiness with his life and a lack of clarity on how to change things.

The first thing that struck me on meeting James was that he was a highly sensitive and empathetic person, and I could see why his business was successful. He spent a lot of time listening to and supporting his clients, and I wondered if he was able to disconnect from them at the end of the day. It was apparent that, as a sensitive person, safety would be a key issue for him, and he wasn't feeling this in his relationship or in his living arrangements.

Applying the FAWA Formula

Applying the 5NNs (*see Chapter 6*) wasn't hard with James as he was so health-savvy but there was some work to be done with his relationship with technology, which had become a comfort and a distraction for him but definitely wasn't helping his sleep. The first thing I advised him to do was to stop measuring his sleep patterns with the phone app (he'd been advised to take some measurements by a doctor at a sleep clinic), to keep electronics out of his bedroom at night and to stop playing computer games in the evening. I also advised him to take breaks away from technology regularly throughout the day.

Even at the first session, because he was so in touch with his body, James was ready to use more advanced tools so we worked on the following techniques from the **Pure Sleep Programme, Deeper Tools II** (*see Chapter 9*):

- Drawing in the Shen to enable him to withdraw from technology, clients and external distractions, and so draw his energy inwards throughout the day (*see page 151*).
- Bedtime yoga – to help calm his nervous system and build safety before sleep (*see page 161*).
- Cutting the cords – to disconnect from worries and clients (*see page 155*).

We also looked some of the ideas in the **Energy for Life Programme** (*see Chapter 11*), and talked about his feelings both at home and in his close relationships, and how to navigate the uncertainties of life.

It was important for James to understand who he was as a human being – his sensitivity and the way he related to other people and his relationship with nature. However, as is often the case in the first session, I didn't want to overwhelm him with too many tools and wanted him to work more specifically on accessing pure healing sleep to increase and stabilise his energy levels. He was in some turmoil as to what to do about his relationship with his girlfriend but I advised him to put any decision-making on hold until he was feeling safer and more grounded in himself – and getting better sleep.

Second Session

James came to see me for his second session six weeks later. Progress had been made. His sleep was much improved, he'd only had one 'bad' night terror and three or four milder nightmares since applying the 5NNs (*see Chapter 6*) and was waking up with good energy. He still experienced moments of anxiety but found that the breathing exercises – 'noticing three exhalations' (*see page 140*) and 'drawing in the Shen' (*see page 151*) – helped a lot and he was making an effort to get out into nature more.

He'd ended his relationship with his girlfriend and was moving out of his flat in a couple of weeks. He said that even though he was feeling a 'sort of loneliness', he was content to be this way for now and felt he had made the right decisions.

Looking back at his notes for the purpose of writing this, I note that I wrote the word 'FLY!!' at the end of the page because this is exactly what I felt James was ready to do.

Two Years Later

I wrote to James to ask his permission to use his story for this book. He replied with some feedback for me:

I am doing good thank you. I've been getting on well and moved into my own house. I feel very settled now, living on my own with my dog Stanley. The night terrors have disappeared and I continue to use the breathing techniques and meditations to this day.

Finding the contentment in small parts of life to keep me settled and grounded! You did a lot for me and I will be forever grateful!

Case Study 2: Finding Safety, Stillness and Self-acceptance

First Session

Nathalie, a 21-year-old university student, came to see me over a year ago. At well over 1.8 metres (6 feet), she had an attractive and sunny disposition. She loved university life and was studying hard for her finals but she'd suffered from night terrors since age 11. Sometimes the terrors were so extreme that she found herself ripping up her bedsheets and hitting her head against the wall.

Coming from a supportive family of high achievers, Nathalie put a lot of pressure on herself to do well, and after getting top grades at school was now studying at one of the most prestigious universities in the UK. However, school hadn't been a positive experience for her, as she had been severely bullied for being so tall and had felt very isolated. She was enjoying university life and had a good circle of friends, although she tended to be the one who supported them rather than an even balance of give and take.

Nathalie was not only extremely intelligent but also highly creative. Often her creativity sprang to life at night and she would stay up all night writing screenplays and designing art sculptures. She felt she achieved her best results when she was 'driving herself into the ground'.

Nathalie suffered from severe tightness in her neck and shoulders, ground her teeth at night and had to wear a mouth guard. She dreaded going to bed and, although she came across as being positive and optimistic, she described her nights as 'hellish' and her bed as 'the enemy'. She often lay in bed feeling depressed and 'not good enough', wondering why she was pushing herself so hard. In desperation she had even called a charity helpline a few times.

Applying the FAWA Formula

Nathalie's eating pattern needed some fine-tuning. I advised her to include more protein in her breakfast cereals (such as nuts) and to avoid caffeine before eating. She was pretty sensible about avoiding caffeine after 2 p.m., but she needed to increase her water intake. The 5NNs (*see Chapter 6*) taken care of, we then talked about a cull on technology after 9 p.m. in the evenings and particularly her tendency to reply to text and social media messages from friends who reached out to her at that time. It was clear to me that she needed to understand her tendency to over-give in her relationships and the boundaries she needed to put in place so that she could sleep. She also needed to be a little more active and was planning to walk more and join a yoga and meditation class.

As with James, I felt Nathalie was ready to engage with some deeper work so I showed her 'breathe deeply' (*see page 24*) as well as 'noticing three exhalations' (*see page 140*) and 'drawing in the Shen' (*see page 151*) exercises from the **Pure Sleep Programme, Deeper Tools II** (*see Chapter 9*) and advised her to use the latter technique at night-time, first thing in the morning and throughout the day in order to help her find stillness and silence.

Second Session

We ended up not seeing each other for another six weeks due to Nathalie sitting exams and I was travelling with business. However, in this time there'd been some significant improvements, as Nathalie reported feeling much calmer and finding getting to sleep easier. She had also only had two night terrors since cleaning up her energy.

She'd moved to a quieter and more comfortable room at her university campus, and this felt good. She was going to a yoga and meditation class and regularly using the breathing techniques that I'd showed her. She was also more aware of what tended to trigger her night terrors: one had occurred after her grandmother had been seriously ill; the other when a friend was going through a distressing time and she'd been offering a lot of support. She was a little unsettled about the uncertainties that lay ahead and we talked about using the mind-set of 'I wonder' from the **Energy for Life Programme** (*see page 203*) rather than 'I hope'. I was thrilled when she said that she saw her night terrors as 'a blessing' (her words) and an opportunity to become more self-aware (*see page 207*).

My notes after this second session read 'Excellent progress' and we agreed that Nathalie would stay in touch and call me if she needed further support, and particularly over the exam period later in the year.

Third Session

Nathalie got in touch 10 months later as her sleep had deteriorated. She was crying out in her sleep, sleeping for a few hours, then waking in the early hours and unable to get back to sleep. She was living in temporary accommodation while she decided on the next steps in her life. She'd done exceptionally well in her exams and had secured a temporary, much-sought-after public engagement at a well-known museum. A great opportunity, but it was high pressure, and on top of this she was about to travel to the US for auditions and interviews for a prestigious fellowship at a top US university. She needed support – I could tell that she was feeling wired and overwhelmed.

During the session it was very clear that Nathalie was running in SURVIVAL mode (*see page 44*). She was eating healthily but this wasn't enough – her mind was in overdrive and running the show with thoughts of what could go wrong, uncertainty and fear about the future and worry about not being good enough. We worked together on the 'grounding and rooting' exercise (*see page 153*) in the **Pure Sleep Programme, Deeper Tools II**, both sitting with our feet planted firmly on the floor and breathing deeply into the belly.

My aim was to help her to slow things right down so that she could see the reality of her situation (which was actually pretty good). The breakthrough came halfway through the session when Nathalie finally allowed herself to feel what she needed to feel and what she'd been running away from all along – fear (*see page 38*). At this point, she started crying and just allowed the tears to flow.

We ended the session talking about coming home regularly (*see page 174*), allowing feelings and trusting herself to know

227

that she has the resources to deal with whatever was coming her way, and trusting that life was supporting her.

One Year Later

A week ago I wrote to Nathalie to ask her permission to use her story for this book. She replied with some feedback:

Professionally, things are going really well. It's an exciting role but there's also a lot of pressure and when things get tough my sleep goes round the bend. However, when that happens, I now have the resources you gave me to tackle it as it comes up.

I am trying to carve out more me time, remembering to breathe deeply and to come home to myself more often. Our conversations have actually been informing my artistic work a lot – one of my big tasks as a director is to hold my space, give myself room to sit back and download moment-to-moment. I'm trying to be less frantic in life and work, and when that is the case, my sleep is so much better. The big learning curve is learning to relax (and enjoy it) – but I suspect that's a lifelong goal.

The good news is that the night terrors side of the equation is on the whole MUCH better – they still pop up when I'm very stressed, but feel it's much more under control, and I try to take them as signs that I need to be making more head space for myself during the day.

It's a case of onwards and upwards, but I feel that what has been in the past a situation of daily struggle against exhaustion is now much more manageable – for which I am very thankful.

Case Study 3: A Shift from Surviving to Thriving

First Session

Tom, a 38-year-old manager, was referred to see me by his company's Human Resources department after sending an extremely career-limiting email to a client at 2 a.m. and, as a result, signed off work with 'stress and work-related anxiety'. A week into his leave, I could see immediately that Tom was wired and jittery, sitting on the edge of his seat and speaking very quickly. For the first half of the session it was hard to get a word in, so I just listened and took notes. He told me about his work history and that although he'd always done well he tended to find himself in situations where he was 'bullied' by overbearing managers.

In his current job he was struggling to get on with his line manager who made him feel as though he wasn't good enough – even though he was working up to 100 hours a week and not getting home until 2 a.m. most days. He'd recently got married but hardly saw his wife, who was increasingly concerned about the long hours he was working and the fact he was drinking heavily in order to relax at the end of the day. He described his energy as 'mostly high but fluctuates dramatically' – he was drinking 10 espressos and three cans of diet cola a day. Tom simply wasn't getting enough sleep and needed to watch TV in bed on his laptop to fall asleep and woke exhausted, needing three alarms to rouse him.

As usual, technology was playing its part here. Tom was never separated from his devices. Even though he'd been signed off work, he constantly checked his emails and social media feeds. He simply couldn't disconnect and slept with two phones and a tablet beside him at night. At work he couldn't concentrate and worked chaotically, multitasking and finding it hard to concentrate.

Tom described his upbringing and family dynamics as 'challenging', with an overprotective mother and 'overbearing and bullying father'. Relationships with siblings were also fraught. Throughout the session I could see shades of Tom's true personality – a bright, lively, funny and creative man – but he didn't feel understood and had been described at work as a 'cartoon character'.

Applying the FAWA Formula

At this initial session, I knew that there was no point in trying to go deeper, as Tom desperately needed to clean up his energy. Several times during the session I had to ask him to stop and lean back in the chair, and so after describing how to use the 5NNs (*see Chapter 6*) I also shared the 'breathe deeply' exercise from Chapter 1 (*see page 24*) and also 'drawing in the Shen' from the **Pure Sleep Programme, Deeper Tools II** (*see Chapter 9*), and he seemed to respond well to both of these exercises. He left the session with the 5 Non-negotiables (*see Chapter 6*) in mind and I invited him to play with the breathing exercises and see how he got on.

Second Session

Tom returned two weeks later saying that he was feeling 'much better'. His energy and demeanour had really shifted and, as he settled back in the chair in my consulting room, he seemed to be in a quiet, contemplative mood. He had made a number of changes, including giving up caffeine totally –

despite 'ferocious' headaches, leaving technology outside the bedroom and not checking emails until he'd eaten breakfast. He was also swimming regularly.

He'd become very aware of what he needed to do in order to feel safe to sleep and was trying to read in the evenings and going to bed earlier. He was finding it hard to pull back from technology but was very aware of when he was using it as an avoidance or distraction strategy. He was regularly using the 'drawing in Shen' exercise (*see page 151*) and, in fact, this was a revelation to him, as he began to notice the difference this simple technique made to his thinking, his energy levels and the choices he was making. He had taken to calling the technique his 'hibiscus moments', as he described the technique as the opening and closing of a flower throughout the day. He aimed to find several hibiscus moments throughout the day, starting with first thing in the day and last thing at night as he drifted off to sleep.

His sleep had improved somewhat and he was getting to sleep easily but he was waking at 2 a.m. and finding it hard to turn his mind off from worrying. I showed him how to calm his heart by using the words 'thank you' from the **Energy for Life Programme** (*see page 158*) – and again this was a revelation to him, and I witnessed yet another shift in his demeanour as this simple but powerful technique took effect.

Completely off his own back, Tom had started reflecting on the relationships and dynamics within his family and had started reading Gary Chapman's *The Five Love Languages*. His wife said he was a 'completely different man'.

Third Session

Again, there were a number of marked improvements and Tom had continued using all the positive strategies and was sleeping better. He was due to return to work in two weeks' time but he wasn't feeling great about this and had noticed that every time he thought about going back he became anxious. An old back problem had flared up and he was now on strong painkillers. He was thinking about leaving the job and was feeling very unsure about the future. Tom was definitely doing The Real Work (*see Chapter 10*).

Over the course of the next six months, Tom wrote to me a few times to update me on his situation. His health and energy levels were much improved and, interestingly, his back problem had virtually disappeared, and this coincided with leaving his job to set up his own business with a friend. With his wife's blessings, he was taking some big risks but was confident about the direction his life was taking.

I received this update a week ago:

> Personally I see myself as a work in progress. I have my off days but have learnt to compartmentalise issues and cut out the things that put me at 95 per cent capacity with no reserve to cope when the big issues arise. I am, it would seem, unmanageable to most people – I'm quite happy with that.
>
> I was thinking I would like to see you, as my business grows the pressure will too. A top-up may be a good investment in me.
>
> So thank you for remembering me, thank you for our time together. You really did save my life!

Different Stories, Common Theme

Each person in the above studies was able to bring about significant shifts in their energy levels, sleep quality and life by making small changes. Their bodies were constantly giving them messages and feedback, and all they had to do was listen. Tom's experience with his back is a particularly powerful illustration of this. In addition,

• Once we listen to our body's innate intelligence and follow its guidance, it becomes stronger and more honed over time.
• Once the initial shifts had taken place – energy balanced and sleep restored – the life force energy then sets us on the right trajectory.

Naturally, not everyone is able to change their lives in this way and there are clients I never see again and know that they haven't been able to shift. And there are people who sit in the auditoriums listening to me, who are often the most cynical and disbelieving, but sometimes these are the ones who have the biggest shifts and then write to tell me about it.

Some people – and thankfully they are a minority – are completely unable to buy into the FAWA formula. Changing habits and behaviours can be tough, and I completely understand this. I also believe that sometimes we need to stay a bit stuck, as there are more lessons to be learnt by staying where we are.

Years ago when I was at university a friend dragged me to a yoga class and I enjoyed it – the feeling of calm was a revelation to me – but I never went again and didn't return to yoga for over 15 years. But maybe if I'd changed my ways then I wouldn't be doing what I'm doing now, and I wouldn't have written this book.

Keep It Simple

I've shared a lot with you in this book – probably more than you expected – but don't be overwhelmed. Take small steps. Keep it simple and allow the 5 Non-negotiables (*see Chapter 6*) to get you started.

- Eat breakfast every day within 30 minutes of rising. Start gently if you have to. Make this a sacred ritual to start your day.
- Drink at least 2 litres (3½ pints) of water a day. Give those 75 trillion cells what they need in order to bring through pure, vibrant energy.
- Reduce or cut out caffeine. Stop over-revving your body and sending it into survival mode.
- Begin an electronic sundown at least 1 hour before you get into bed.
- Aim to get at least four pre-midnight sleeps per week. Be mindful of the vulnerable childlike state that you enter around 10 p.m. Pull your energy inwards. Withdraw from stimulation. Listen to what your body and soul need in order to feel safe. Be peaceful. Be gentle. Rest and prepare to sleep.

And if you're ready for it, use the two most powerful words in the dictionary as you turn your lights out, if you awaken during the night and upon rising to start your day:

THANK YOU!

Then allow the magic to unfold.

Conclusion

Flying and Flourishing

'My mission in life is not merely to survive, but to thrive; and to do so with some passion, some compassion, some humor, and some style.'

Maya Angelou

You may have come to *Fast Asleep, Wide Awake* due to a sleep problem or because you were exhausted. I hope you've got more than you bargained for and have discovered more than just a solution to your insomnia. I've always known that resolving sleep issues goes way beyond learning to sleep deeply: it's more about initiating a process. A process through which we can begin to access our body's intelligence and potential to connect with a universal wisdom, often referred to as the universal consciousness.

Sleep – when it is sattvic – is a conduit for accessing this universal wisdom.

When you start doing The Real Work I promise you will start to reconnect with a part of yourself that has been underfed and undernourished. Sonia Choquette, a dynamic spiritual teacher, aptly describes this in her book *Trust Your*

Vibes as 'psychic anorexia'. Have you been starving yourself? And if so, what do you need to do now to nourish your spirit and soul? Do you know what your spirit wants to be fed?

By asking these questions and paying attention to the answers you will start to plug into a vibrant life force energy, which will enable you to thrive. As young children, we knew what fed our souls and how to tap into vibrant energy. We knew how to be happy, joyful and playful, but somewhere along the line we forgot. And when this goes on for too long the body, cleverly, looks for ways to tell us to wake up and smell the coffee (excuse the pun).

I hope that by now you have found a new way of regarding your amazing body, a new way of listening to it and, most of all, a new way of caring for it. If you have, you are well on your way to a wondrous journey. This journey unfolds in different ways for each of us, but it enables us all to move from merely enduring and surviving life to truly living it.

We each have a responsibility to choose how we want to be in this world and how we co-create our world. Do you want to settle for just surviving and running on fear, busyness and overwhelm? Or you do want more – a life of gratitude, love, compassion and safety – one that our children deserve too? So, as life and technology continually draw us outwards, close your eyes and draw yourself inwards – even just for a moment – and find out who you truly are.

I'll ask you again, what is it that your spirit needs? How does it want to be nourished? Revisit your childhood memories. What made you feel joyful, carefree, silly and light? Who were you at your best? This is what your life force energy is about.

Are you unstoppable, passionate, tempestuous, fiery and commanding? Or are you gentle, sweet, caring and creative? Tune in and remember who you are. When did you last feel like this? And what were you doing?

Therein lies the key to what you need to be doing in order to be flying and flourishing.

Endnotes

1. Bernardi, L. *et al*. 'Cardiovascular, cerebrovascular, and respiratory changes induced by different types of music in musicians and non-musicians: the importance of silence', *Heart*, 92(4) (2006), pp. 445–52; doi:10.1136/hrt.2005.064600.
2. Kirste, I. *et al*. 'Is silence golden? Effects of auditory stimuli and their absence on adult hippocampal neurogenesis', *Brain Structure and Function*, 220(2) (2015), pp. 1221–8.
3. I arrived at these five strategies after many years of working with driven, impatient and exhausted corporate employees who needed effective and practical solutions – and fast. I distilled what would have taken me at least two days to deliver in a lecture to undergraduate physiology students and created a programme that could engage a hungry audience in about 30 minutes. I called them my '5 Non-negotiables' (5NNs) because I'm not particularly imposing, at just over 1.5 metres (5 foot) tall, and can appear gentle and softly spoken, so I needed to use powerful language to sell my message. Calling my five strategies non-negotiable was a way of getting the point across quickly and in a way that didn't invite too much resistance.
4. Korotkov, K. *et al*. 'Application of electrophoton capture (EPC) analysis based on gas discharge visualization (GDV) technique in medicine: A systematic review', *The Journal of Alternative and Complementary Medicine*, 16(1) (2010), pp. 13–25; doi:10.1089/acm.2008.0285.

5. Schulz, H. and Peretz, L. (eds), *Ultradian Rhythms in Physiology and Behavior*, Springer-Verlag, 1985, pp. 11–31.
6. Kirste, I. *et al.* 'Is silence golden? Effects of auditory stimuli and their absence on adult hippocampal neurogenesis', *Brain Structure and Function*, 220(2) (2015), pp. 1221–8.
7. Nedergaard, M. *et al.* 'Sleep drives metabolite clearance from the adult brain', *Science*, 342 (6156) (2013), pp. 373–7, doi: 10.1126/science.1241224.
8. Loomis, A. *et al.* 'Cerebral states during sleep as studied by human brain potentials', *Experimental Psychology*, 21(2) (1937), pp. 127–44.
9. Dement, W. *et al.* 'Cyclic variations in EEG during sleep and their relation to eye movements, body motility, and dreaming', *Electroencephalography and Clinical Neurophysiology*, a, 9(4) (1957), pp. 673–90.
10. Perlis, M. *et al.* 'Beta/Gamma EEG activity in patients with primary and secondary insomnia and good sleeper controls', *Sleep*, 24(1) (2001), pp. 110–17.
11. Rechtschaffen, A. *et al.* (1999). 'Effects of method, duration, and sleep stage on rebounds from sleep deprivation in the rat', *Sleep*, 22 (1) (1999), pp. 11–31.
12. Batterink, L. *et al.* 'Sleep facilitates learning a new linguistic rule', *Neuropsychologia*, 65 (2014), pp. 169–79.
13. Marquié, J. *et al.* Chronic effects of shift work on cognition: findings from the VISAT longitudinal study, *Occup. Environ. Med.*, 72(4) (2015), pp. 258–64.
14. Jan-Dijk, D. *et al.* 'Mistimed sleep disrupts circadian regulation of the human transcriptome', *PNAS*, 111 (2014), E682–91.
15. Thakur, N. and Sharma, D. 'Full moon and crime', *British Medical Journal*, 289 (1984), pp. 22–9.
16. http://www.bbc.co.uk/news/health-25812422; accessed 3 August 2015.
17. https://www.consumerreports.org/cro/2015/03/the-truth-about-sleeping-pills/index.htm; accessed 26 April 2016.

18. Gerber, R. *Vibrational Medicine for the 21st Century*, William Morrow, 2000.

19. http://www.health.harvard.edu/blog/mindfulness-meditation-helps-fight-insomnia-improves-sleep-201502187726; accessed 22 March 2016.

20. http://archinte.jamanetwork.com/article.aspx?articleid=2110998; accessed 22 March 2016.

21. http://www.todaysdietitian.com/newarchives/100112p76.shtml; accessed 22 March 2016.

22. Myss, C. *Anatomy of the Spirit*, Bantam, 1997, pp. 94–283.

23. Jan-Dijk, D. *et al.* 'Mistimed sleep disrupts circadian regulation of the human transcriptome', *PNAS*, 2014; 111: E682–91

24. https://www.psychologytoday.com/blog/brain-wise/201209/why-were-all-addicted-texts-twitter-and-google; accessed 26 April 2016.

25. http://abcnews.go.com/Health/cell-phones-give-brain-burst-caffeine-energy/story?id=2112186; accessed 16 April 2016.

26. http://onlinelibrary.wiley.com/doi/10.1111/j.1365-2869.2008.00718.x/full; accessed 16 April 2016.

27. http://www.ukhypnosis.com/2009/06/17/emile-coues-method-of-%E2%80%9Cconscious-autosuggestion%E2%80%9D/; accessed 24 March 2016.

28. https://www.psychologytoday.com/blog/feeling-it/201309/20-scientific-reasons-start-meditating-today; accessed 22 March 2016.

29. http://www.bps.org.uk/news/bps-journal-paper-insomnia-and-control-emotion; accessed 22 March 2016.

30. Dwoskin, H. and Canfield, C. *The Sedona Method*, Sedona Press, 2008.

31. Seligman, M. E. P. *Authentic Happiness*, Free Press, 2002.

32. Hamilton, D. *Why Kindness Is Good for You*, Hay House, 2010.

33. Wood, A. *et al.* 'Gratitude influences sleep through the mechanism of pre-sleep cognitions', *Psychosomatic Research*, 66(1) (2009), pp. 43–8.

34. Bennett, M. and Lengacher, C. 'Humor and laughter may influence health. IV. Humor and immune function', *Evidence-Based Complementary and Alternative Medicine*, 6(2) (2009), pp. 159–64.

35. Lighta, C. *et al.* 'More frequent partner hugs and higher oxytocin levels are linked to lower blood pressure and heart rate in premenopausal women', *Biological Psychology*, 69 (2005), pp. 5–21.

36. Jobst, K. *et al.* 'Diseases of meaning, manifestations of health and metaphor', *Alternative and Complementary Medicine – Research on Paradigm, Practice and Policy*, 5(6) (1999), pp. 495–502.

Bibliography

Bloom, William, *Feeling Safe*, Piatkus, 2007

Chopra, Deepak, *Creating Health*, Mariner Books, 1995

Choquette, Sonia, *Trust Your Vibes*, Hay House, 2004

Covey, Stephen, *The Seven Habits of Highly Effective People*, Simon & Schuster, 2004

Damasio, Antonio, *The Feeling of What Happens*, Vintage, 2000

Emmons, Robert A. and McCullough, Michael E., *The Psychology of Gratitude*, OUP USA, 2004

Hamilton, David, *Why Kindness Is Good for You*, Hay House, 2010

Honoré, Carl, *In Praise of Slow*, Orion, 2005

Lazarus, Jeremy, *Ahead of the Game*, Ecademy Press, 2006

O'Donohue, John, *Anam Cara*, Harper Perennial, 1998

Ramachandran, V.S. and Blakeslee, Sandra, *Phantoms in the Brain*, Fourth Estate, 1999

Stiffelman, Susan, *Parenting with Presence*, New World Library, 2015

Turkle, Sherry, *Alone Together*, Basic Books, 2013

Wren, Barbara, *Cellular Awakening*, Hay House, 2009

Resources

Complementary Medicine

The College of Naturopathic Medicine: http://www.
naturopathy-uk.com/
British Homeopathic Association: http://www.
britishhomeopathic.org/
The Association of Traditional Chinese Medicine and
Acupuncture UK: http://www.atcm.co.uk/
The British Complementary Medicine Association: http://
www.bcma.co.uk/
The Association of Natural Medicine: http://www.
associationnaturalmedicine.co.uk/
The British Medical Acupuncture Society: http://www.
medical-acupuncture.co.uk/
The British Acupuncture Council: http://www.acupuncture.
org.uk/
The Association of Reflexologists: http://www.aor.org.uk/

Sleep and Wellness

www.sensitivesleepers.com
www.netdoctor.co.uk

Yoga and Meditation

The British Wheel of Yoga: http://www.bwy.org.uk/
The British Meditation Society: http://www.
   britishmeditationsociety.org/
The Mindfulness Association: http://www.
   mindfulnessassociation.org/

Therapy and Counselling

The British Association for Counselling and Psychotherapy:
   http://www.bacp.co.uk/

Index